FLEXIBLE STEEL

By Jon Engum, Master RKC

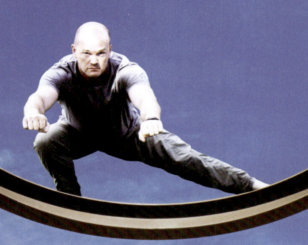

An Insider's Guide to Ultimate Flexibility

FLEXIBLE STEEL

AN INSIDER'S GUIDE TO ULTIMATE FLEXIBILITY

By Jon Engum, Master RKC

© Copyright 2013, Jon Engum
A Dragon Door Publications, Inc. production
All rights under International and Pan-American Copyright conventions.
Published in the United States by: Dragon Door Publications, Inc.
5 East County Rd B, #3 • Little Canada, MN 55117
Tel: (651) 487-2180 • Fax: (651) 487-3954
Credit card orders: 1-800-899-5111 • Email: support@dragondoor.com • Website: www.dragondoor.com

ISBN 10: 0-938045-97-0   ISBN 13: 978-0-938045-97-7
This edition first published in January, 2013
Printed in China

No part of this book may be reproduced in any form or by any means without the prior written consent of the Publisher, excepting brief quotes used in reviews.

Book design and cover by Derek Brigham • www.dbrigham.com • (763) 208-3069 • bigd@dbrigham.com

DISCLAIMER: The author and publisher of this material are not responsible in any manner whatsoever for any injury that may occur through following the instructions contained in this material. The activities, physical and otherwise, described herein for informational purposes only, may be too strenuous or dangerous for some people and the reader(s) should consult a physician before engaging in them.

Table of Contents

1. Introduction 1
2. Who Needs Rotation? 5
3. The Three Big S's 7
4. Get Your Kicks…Up! 9
5. From Tin Man To Plastic Man 13
6. The Tactical Frog 39
7. Splits Defined 47
8. Stemming Your Way To The Splits 49
9. Front Splits For Back Health 55
10. Just Add Water 61
11. Escape Your Fighting Stance 65

Resources 71

About the Author 73

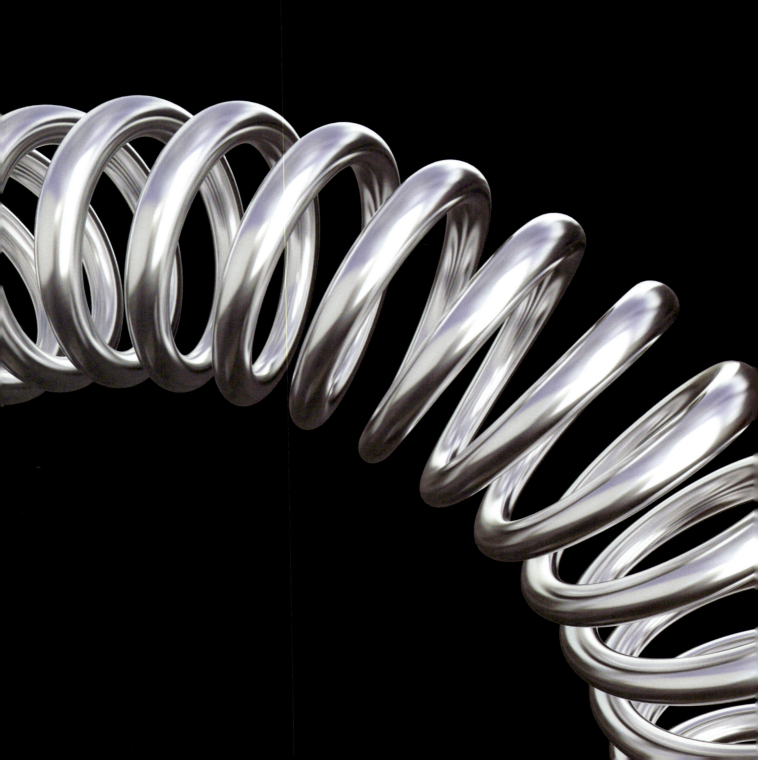

Dedicated
To my Michelle,
without you nothing
would be possible.

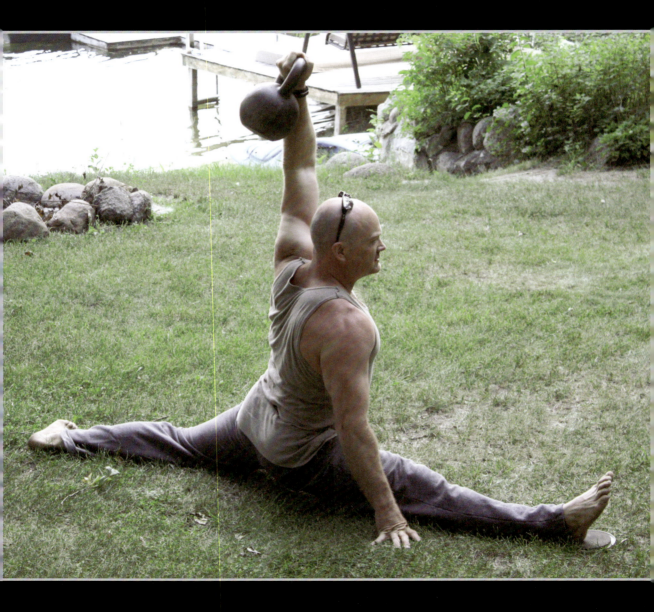

Foreword to Flexible Steel

By Mark Reifkind, Master RKC

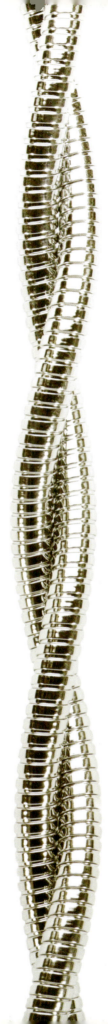

First off, Jon Engum is the Real Deal. Let's get that out of the way quickly. To me there is no greater compliment. In a world of 'personal trainers' who don't have time to exercise because they are 'working' too much, Jon Engum walks his talk. And has for over 30 years.

Last I looked, they don't hand out 7th Degree Black Belts and the title Grandmaster to dabblers. Jon has been training, competing, studying and teaching Tae Kwan Do for all those 30 years.

That should be enough for anyone, but Jon also holds 4th degree Black Belts in Hapkido and Kumdo/Kumbup (Sword). Oh yes, and he is also a Master RKC instructor.

He holds, like myself, a PhD from the School of Hard Knocks.

And is still one of the nicest, humblest and competent men you will ever meet.

I have had the honor and privilege of working with and watching Jon teach at RKC certifications for the last 6 years. And every time I am more and more impressed with his skills, his techniques, his curiosity for all things training and strength related and his ability to communicate those things to his students.

Like all great teachers he is the perpetual student, never resting in his quest for a deeper understanding of techniques and subtleties to further his abilities as well as his charges.

This fantastic book is direct evidence of that quest.

I have more than a passing interest in flexibility and have for over 40 years. It began in 1972 when I became a competitive gymnast and continues to this day as I continue to recover and regain abilities lost from those 40 years of training and competition in various sports.

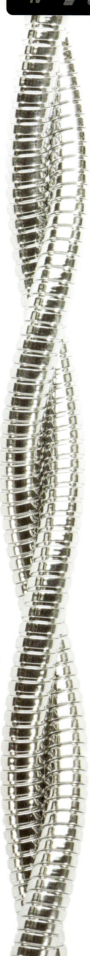

Having been in the game all those years, I have seen all the fitness trends come and go. Flexibility training went from being completely ignored, to being given a passing nod in the realm of the 'functional training' fad, to being upstaged again of late, as "mobility" becomes the buzzword of the day.

As a Real Deal athlete that has to put it all on the line every time he steps on to the mat to fight, Jon knows that without enough real flexibility to get his leg easily to his opponent's head, mobility won't be enough.

He realized this the hard way when he woke up one day and realized he had less flexibility than his beginning students. An 'aha" moment to say the least. The difference is that Jon figured out how to solve that problem, and we, the readers and his students, are the beneficiaries of that study.

He is more flexible and mobile than when he was a teenager and strong as a bull as well. And he is no small guy either. At 200 lbs of solid muscle I found out the easy way why no one would want to be kicked by this man.

Jon was taking the Bodyweight Exercise Workshop taught by Pavel, myself and Senior RKC, Max Shank in 2011 and was working on his handstand, a fairly new skill to him. Throwing himself into the process with the perfect 'beginners mind' he listened to my instructions carefully as I prepared to spot him as he kicked up to a free handstand.

He kicked with his lead leg, as instructed, and let it float until I could grab it as he approached the upside down position. What I didn't expect was that his leg felt like it was made from a serious BIG chunk of hardwood and as dense as well. It almost knocked me off my feet just from a casual push off to get to a handstand!

I can only imagine what that might feel like if he directed it with full force into a guy's rib cage! With his effortless flexibility and ease of movement one would never know his legs are that heavy and strong. **Flexible Steel**, indeed.

Again, Jon not only teaches, it he lives it.

This book is a simple one, but don't let that fool you. The drills and techniques inside look like many things you might have seen before, but the details make all the difference.

Jon deconstructs stretching and flexibility and makes it a very simple plan to follow. Simple, not easy. As all great things are ☺. Jon takes some old methods and does them one better—allowing you to make quantum leaps forward in your flexibility and useable strength. He also shows us his own unique approach to getting into some serious splits in the fastest time possible.

I like to say it's all easy til it's heavy. Jon would say, it's all easy til you have to do the splits. And he'd be right.

And that's where this book really shines, in Jon's detailed analysis of the splits—and how he mastered them and how you can too. In the process, he opened up the rest of his body and regained a youthful flexibility and mobility that we all would love to possess.

This book is not only for martial artists and gymnasts, but for everybody that wants or needs a more flexible, supple body and the movement and health that come along with that.

Awesome job Jon, so glad to know you and call you friend.

Mark Reifkind
Master RKC

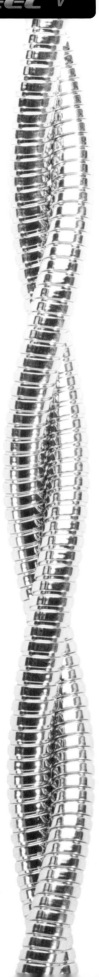

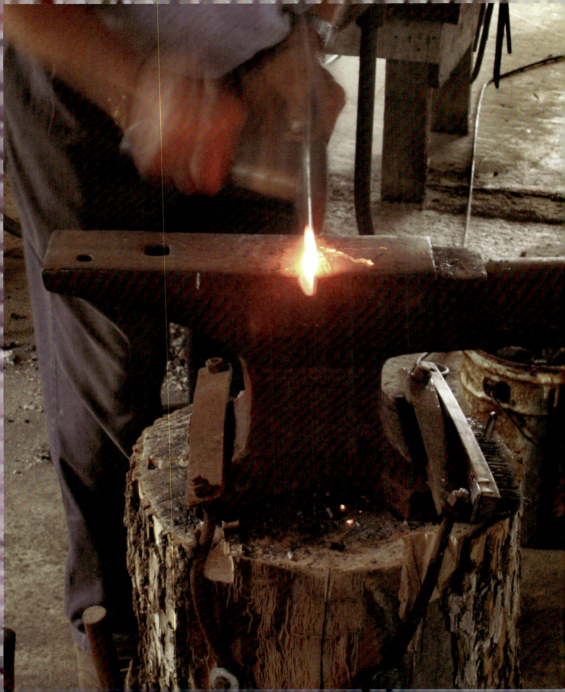

Chapter 1

Introduction

Flexible Steel
An Insider's Guide to Ultimate Flexibility

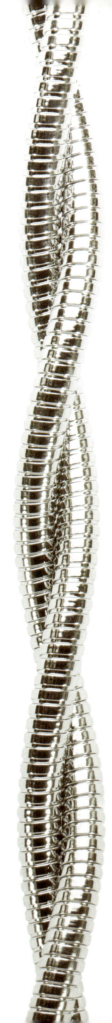

As a young boy running through the streets of town on my way to Taekwondo, I'm pretty sure my feet weren't touching the ground. For me, the passion was always there. I earned my first black belt in 1984 and have always been teaching to some degree since then. It is all I have ever done, it is all I know. Today I feel fortunate to be a martial arts instructor.

Before—and for quite some time after opening my own school—I was a very active tournament competitor. Sparring was my game and I managed to find a tournament to compete in almost every weekend. It's what I did for fun; little did I know I was turning into something like a rodeo cowboy. We've all heard the stories of rodeo cowboys going from town to town on the circuit, with broken down pickup trucks and even more broken down bodies. That was me, although I was fighting, not busting broncos—training during the week and fighting on weekends, week after week.

In the early days I had no idea how to peak for a competition or cycle my training. My training cycle, if you can call it such, went something like this: Monday = Hard training, Tuesday = Harder Training, Wednesday = Damn Hard Training, Thursday = "F"ing Hard Training, Friday = Travel, Saturday = Compete, Sunday = come home and try to figure out how to train around the injuries received on Saturday.

Not that this was that unusual. Martial artists were relatively a small segment of society back then and no one had the smarts to put sports science into play…Hell, we were not "athletes" we were fighters. Most everyone was doing things the same as I was—well at least the cats I was competing against.

I had some success along the way winning more often than not and I managed to rack up some state and national titles. But in the process I was destroying my body. The natural resilience of youth can only go so far. To take the cowboy analogy a little further, they often talk of a used and abused horse as being "ridden hard and put away wet." Well, I was becoming that broken down horse.

I began to notice that during my training I was becoming stiffer and stiffer. I would wake up in the morning like the proverbial "Tin Man" with aching, tight muscles and creaking, rusty joints.

This constant state of deterioration was really driven home to me when new students would come into class and naturally display more flexibility and more mobility than my "professionally" trained body. Can you imagine the disgrace I felt as the "Master"? More like Master Tin Man.

There comes a turning point in one's life when you have a blinding flash of the obvious and this was mine…what I was doing was not only **not** working but I was actually sabotaging my own efforts in the name of self-improvement. So I decided to take the bull by the horns (cowboy pun intended). I needed better technology than just toughness. Because Martial Arts was my profession, I was unhindered by a "real" job and able to dedicate the time needed to truly become a "seeker of flexibility truth." I went to every stretching guru or workshop I could find, no matter the expense or distance.

What did I discover? The flexibility world is running rampant with charlatans.

The flexibility scene offers up more false gods than a TV evangelist with a crack habit. One guy would say do this and that and in six months you will gain a few inches in your stretch. Or take this supplement "snake oil" twice a day for a year and you will miraculously be able to do the splits.

It was about this time that I received a magazine in the mail, about this tough Russian guy, Pavel Tsatsouline. He was promising all kinds of gains in what at the time seemed like over-the-top marketing. We all remember the old adage, if it seems too good to be true it probably is. But I was on a quest and had already experienced the good, the bad and the ugly. I have always been of the mind that if I can take one

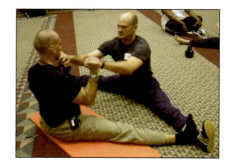

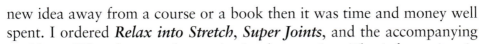

new idea away from a course or a book then it was time and money well spent. I ordered *Relax into Stretch*, *Super Joints*, and the accompanying videos. What happened next is simply amazing. The information in these products delivered more then they promised—and they promised a lot. My gains and movement ability begin to come back, and that was just the beginning. I thought, if the information in the books could deliver like this, what would it be like to actually train with this guy…I signed up for Pavel's next seminar and needless to say I was not disappointed.

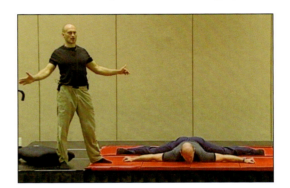

Now, I was used to getting the "try this and this and stick to it for several months and you will see improvement"…not with Pavel. The man had me in the splits that day, something I could never do in the past. The results were instant and remarkable.

**Pavel's comment: "Jon, if you think that is cool, you have to check out kettlebells."
And the rest is history.**

The following pages are my interpretation of my acquired bit of stretching knowledge and experimentation. It is my hope to show you how to combine the knowledge gained in the works such as *Relax Into Stretch* and *Super Joints* as well as some homegrown stretching advice gleaned over the course of my journey. It goes without saying that if you have not read the works mentioned above, STOP and order them immediately. They will be referenced heavily here and you simply cannot be without them.

I hope you practice and enjoy the tips and techniques that are offered up in the following pages and that they breathe new life into you as they have for me.

I stand today more flexible than I was in my teens and 20s. I achieved the full splits for the first time in my life around the age of forty, and if I can do it then you can too.

"Knowledge is a journey not a destination!"

Jon Engum

Jon Engum

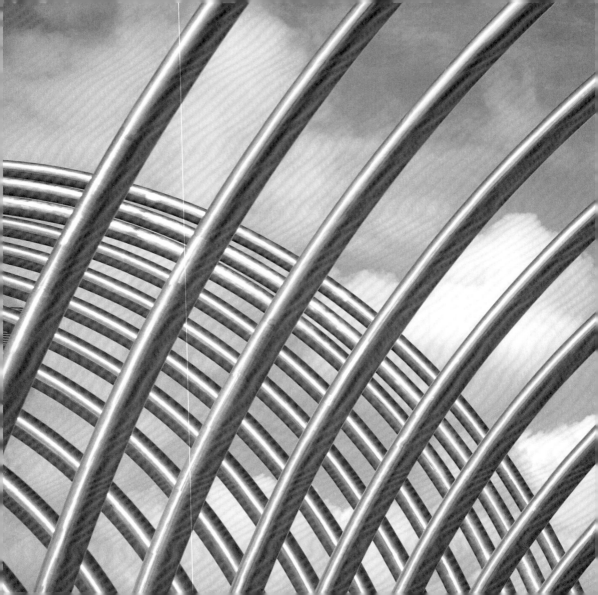

CHAPTER 2

Who Needs Rotation?

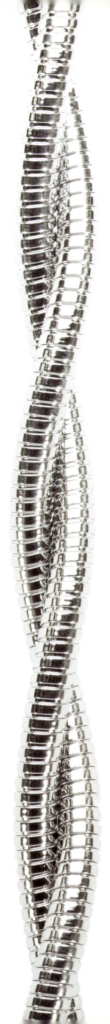

Anyone who plays a sport that demands rotational power and mobility. Think about it. If you play golf, tennis, baseball, or the martial arts, what would an extra 12 inches of pain-free twist do for the enjoyment and performance of your game? As a matter of fact, I can't think of a single person that would not benefit from this extra freedom of rotational movement.

Maybe the closest thing to a sport you play is being a soccer mom driving your kids around. Well, this one tip could actually save your life and the lives of your kids. Ever have a close call while driving because you lacked the mobility to comfortably look over your shoulder for oncoming traffic?

Say goodbye to that problem forever! You will virtually have eyes in the back of your head after doing just 3 simple steps.

1. Stand erect.

2. Feet flat on the ground and lock your knees. Do not bend them throughout the rest of this drill, or else.

3. Without moving your feet, rotate your upper body as far as you can to the right.

When you have achieved your greatest rotation, pick out an object with your eyes at maximum rotation and memorize it.

We have just established a base line of your rotation.

Next, you will retest this move—but this time you will focus on three things while you turn.

1. Contract your left glute or cheek, not the ones on your face either. I mean really contract it, to the point of cramping.

2. At the same time try to drive your left heel through the ground. I want to see an indentation when you are done.

3. I want you to imagine that the front of your left hip—kind of where your pocket would be—is getting longer. Do all three steps while slowly turning as you retest.

If you followed the directions you should easily add 6-7 inches to your previous score!

You will retest one more time doing all of the above plus three more things.

1. Imagine that your body is being hoisted in the air by your neck. In other words try to get as tall and elongated as possible.

2. Visualize space being made between each vertebra.

3. Starting at your tailbone, in your mind, sequentially rotate each vertebra. When you get as far as you possibly can, I want you to rotate seven more imaginary vertebrae, as if your backbone kept extending above your head.

Check out where your starting point was and now where your new max is—most people have gained 12 inches or more!

Magic? No!

You have just applied the 3 fundamental S's to a stretch. For more on this, read on.

By the way, make sure you do the other side or you may be walking in a circle the rest of the day.

Did you get some amazing results? Are you considering changing your name to Linda Blair? Old movie reference, sorry.

CHAPTER 3

The Three Big S's Of Stretching

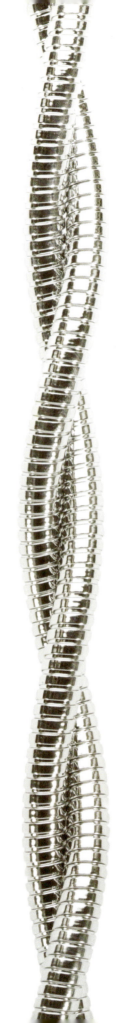

When I teach at a live stretching event, I like to lead off with the rotational movement drill because it illustrates the three main principles of power stretching a.k.a. **The Three S's**. Once you understand the Three S's you can apply them to not only any stretching exercise but also to any movement... be it martial arts, dance, or even strength training.

"Give a man a fish and you feed him for a day. Teach a man to fish and you feed him for a lifetime." Old Chinese Proverb

So let's learn how to "fish"...

S1 = Strength

The first S is for Strength. Use strength in your movements. Do not just yield to gravity or passively move into stretch but actively use your muscles to pull or push you into positions.

I am not talking about going faster, but actively using muscular force to get you where you want to go.

Example: In the rotational drill, from here on out referred to as the "Exorcist", we contract the left glute and drive our left heel into the ground when we are turning to the right.

S2 = Space

The second S stands for Space. Make space inside the body itself. Instead of trying to jam one joint into another, it is much more effective to put them in some traction and literally create some extra room.

In the *Exorcist*, we used this in two different ways. First I told you to visualize the front of your hip getting longer; second I said to imagine that your body was being hoisted in the air by your neck. We were putting your spine into traction in order to create some more space.

More space = greater range of movement

S3 = Spread

Last but not least, the third S is for Spread. As in spread the load. Instead of trying to twist or turn or move from one spot or one joint, try to spread the movement over as many joints and muscles as possible, taking up slack where you can. If you gain a little bit here and a little bit there, it adds up to huge gains.

During our rotational experiment I told you to sequentially rotate each vertebra, starting at your tailbone and working your way up and past your head...spreading the load over your entire spine.

There it is. You have the Keys to the Stretching Kingdom. Apply these to all of your movement needs and reap the rewards.

Still want more? You got it!

Read on to find out how to get your kicks...up.

By the way, I did not invent or systemize the Three S's. They came from Pavel Tsatsouline's work. I am only giving you my take on things... If you have not read *Relax into Stretch* yet, you have homework. If you have, then reread it.

CHAPTER 4

Get Your Kicks...UP!

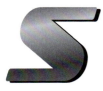coring a perfect head kick is one of the best feelings in the world. The fighting game is much like Christmas...It is much better to give than to receive.

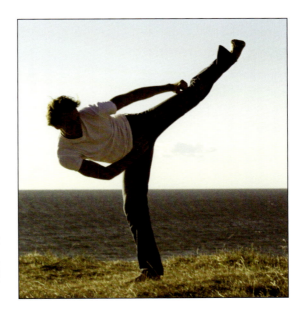

There is no better gift than a well delivered kick to the head, from the kicker's point of view, anyway. This chapter will have a distinct martial arts flavor but even if you have no interest in high kicking, bear with me for a minute and I will bring it around.

In the last chapter, when we were talking about the Three S's to power stretching, I said the first S stands for strength. Interestingly enough, often times it is not lack of flexibility that prevents one from being able to kick high, but lack of strength.

Let's talk about the different types of stretching and I'll give you a cool low-tech, high-concept drill to get your kicks...up.

But before we can get into the hows of combining stretching with strength specifically to improve the height of your kick, let's define different forms of flexibility.

Passive-Static Flexibility

This is what most people are talking about when they say stretching. You are just sitting there stretching...think a toe touch, a sit and reach, or a split. You are using gravity or the weight of your body to stretch. Think relaxed stretching.

Active-Static Flexibility

This is when you are using your own power to move into a stretch, although not with speed. You use the strength of the opposite muscle group—read muscle-agonists—to move into and hold the stretch.

A simple example would be contracting the biceps to stretch the triceps.

Dynamic Flexibility

Just like the name implies, you use dynamic movement to stretch...different types of leg swings, arm swings etc.

The movements start out low and slow and gradually become fast and high. The focus is not on how high you can swing your leg, but how high you can swing your leg while staying loose and relaxed.

Isometric Stretching

This is a power tool and we'll talk about it later.

Okay, so you "just wanna get my kicks up higher." Well here's how.

Dynamic Stretches

Start by doing a few sets of leg swings. A set will consist of 8-12 reps per leg. Do swings to the front, side and back. Remember to start slow and low and work up to high and fast.

Everyone is different, so "high" is what is high for you. Also try to increase the speed from slow to sport speed by the last rep.

Chase the leg swings down with a shot of…

Active-Static Stretching

In the book *Super Joints* by Pavel Tsatsouline, there is a side bar that tells about a Russian kickboxing coach using a form of passive-active stretching to get his fighters' kicks up.

Pavel himself has told me this part of his book is often overlooked…maybe because it is in a sidebar, who knows, but it is powerful.

I will explain it from memory, but I suggest getting *Super Joints* to read the original text.

The coach would have his fighters put their leg up on a platform or table that was just about at their flexibility limit. For a front kick, toes pointed up—for a sidekick or roundhouse, toes sideways.

The fighter would then just chill in that position for a while until his leg relaxed. Next, the fighter would lift his leg up using his own leg power and then the coach would quickly slip a stack of books under his foot allowing him to relax in this new range of movement (ROM).

The process is repeated until the fighter cannot get his leg up any higher. Talk about increasing strength and flexibility at the same time.

The downside of this method is that it really takes two people to pull it off.

Never fear, gentle reader, because I have a solution for all you lone stretchers out there.

Enter the Pulley System

Martial Artists have been using the rope and pulley to stretch their legs since before the front kick was invented. Let's just say it is nothing new, but how I am going to have you use it may just breathe some new life into this low tech apparatus.

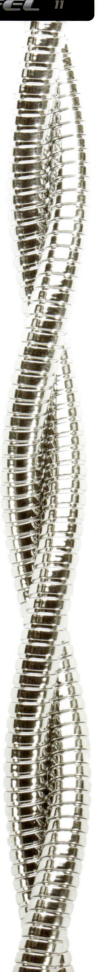

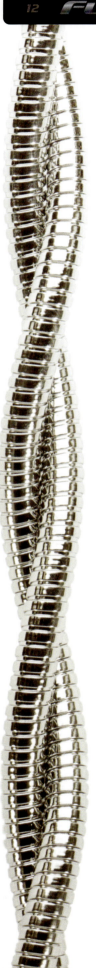

In case you have never experienced this, here is how it is typically done.

Standard "Lame" Method

1. Go to the hardware store and get a pulley and a length of rope.

2. Attach the pulley to the ceiling and thread the rope through the pulley.

3. Tie a loop on one end of the rope. Try an overhead knot on a bight not a hangman's noose.

4. Put foot in loop and pull on the other end of the rope. Leg goes up and you stretch.

Are you thinking that you could have figured that out yourself? But wait...here is the secret!

New Improved Method

Instead of using the rope to lift your leg—passively stretching, use your leg muscles, strength (**S1**) to lift your leg and only use the pulley and rope to take up the slack.

Now you have turned this into an active-passive stretch and you are building specific strength and flexibility at the same time.

About 3 sets of 5 reps - with the reps being the leg lifting part, is about right. You can now do the Russian kickboxer's drill without a training partner.

CHAPTER 5

From The Tin Man to Plastic Man Mobility Drills

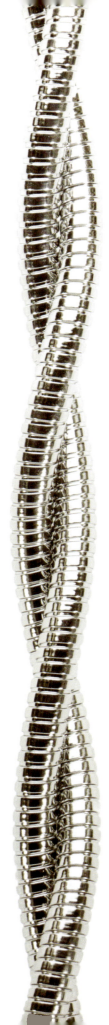

One of the most common limiting factors for most people as they grow older are achy, creaky joints. I will readily admit that the splits may not be everyone's cup of tea, so let's start by talking about something that is a must for everyone, mobility drills.

Mobility drills will lube up your joints and help you to fix damaged ones. These are light movements and rotations designed to take the joints through a full range of movement. Mobility drills are performed as a stand-alone workout in the morning and done for as many reps as you are old and/or can be done before a workout for reps of 10-20.

The term "Mobility Training" was coined by Russian scientist Nikolay Amosov. Amosov claims mobility training can slow down or reverse arthritis. Amosov also formulated the theory of limit loads, which states "The human organism has a great ability to regenerate itself through intense use." The bottom line is to do your mobility drills—they will wake you up better than a shot of double espresso.

You may think of your mobility practice as both a morning recharge and a way to get rid of the "rust" that has accumulated in your joints. Some of you may know the joints themselves do not really have blood flowing to them so the only way to get rid of the waste products or excuse me, crud, that is present in the joints is to bathe them with synovial fluid. The way to get more synovial fluid to the joints is through movement. "Use it or lose it" is not just a cute catch phrase but a hard, cold fact of life when it comes to joint health.

Generally start from your head and work your way down to your feet. The following is one of my recharge series. It has its roots in many different programs, to use a phrase by Master RKC, Jeff O'Connor "Most everything I teach has been stolen from someone I *respect*." This series has a little bit of everything in it. In the immortal words of Bruce Lee "Take what is useful and discard the rest." And that is just what I have done with this series of drills. I have distilled out all of the fluff and only left in the big bang for your training buck movements. I receive lots of positive feedback every time I present this series at a workshop and am always asked to write it up, so here it comes.

Series 1: Standing

1. Forward and Backward Neck Bends—The Yes Movement

Not only are you to nod you head up and down, but try to elongate your whole back from the tail bone to the crown of your head.

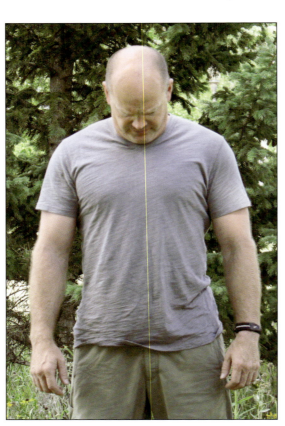
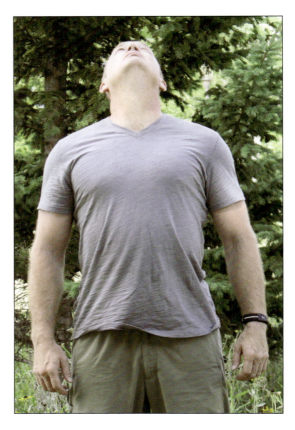

2. Side to Side Neck Bends—The No Movement
Try to see the same spot behind you each way.

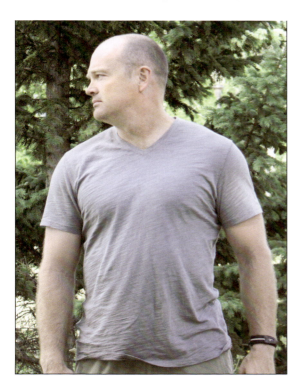
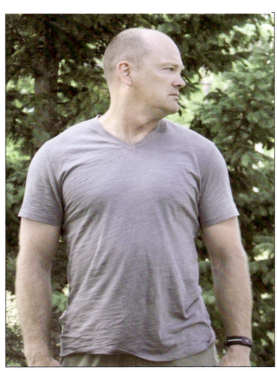

3. Neck Tilts—Jaw to Sky Movements
Try to tilt your head strictly sideways.

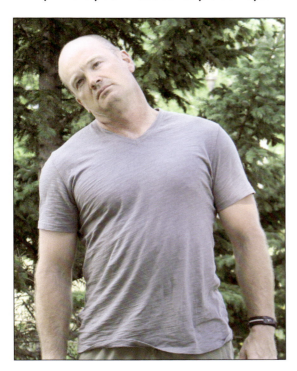
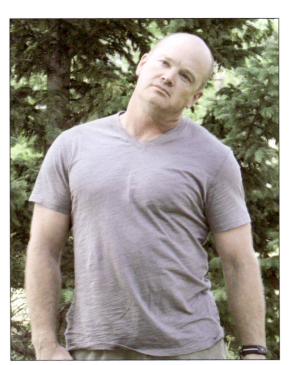

4. Figure of 8's

Trace figure of 8's with your nose "Stevie Wonder" style not "Bewitched".

5. Wrist Circles

Make circular motions first with your palms together then apart. Make sure you go both forward and backward.

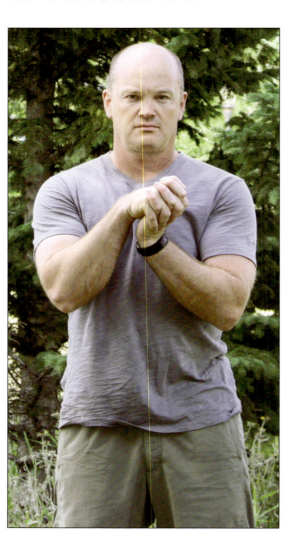
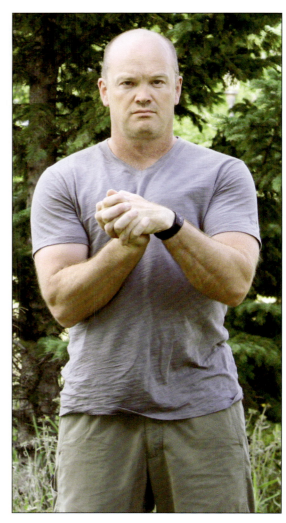

6. Elbow Circles

Place your arms out at about a 45-degree angle, with the point of your elbows down and the pits of your elbows up. Imagine you are trying to put on a pair of sunglasses and miss. Rotate your elbows and wind up back in the starting position. Reverse and repeat.

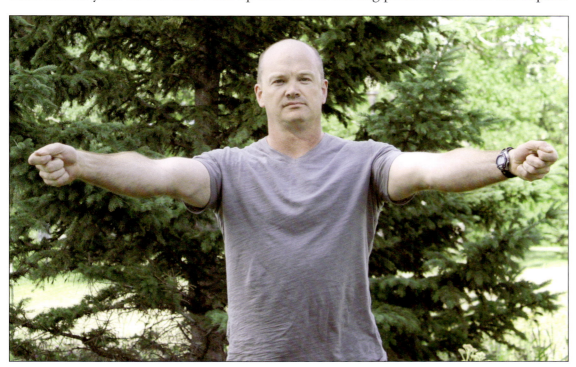

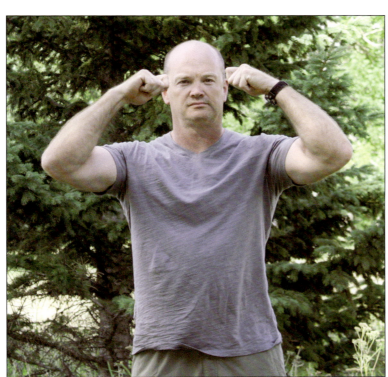

7. Inside elbow circles (Breast Stroke Like Movements)

Single arm, then both arms together. Brush your fingers and the back of your hand on your arm pits. Then try to point straight behind you as if someone is trying to twist your arm behind your back.

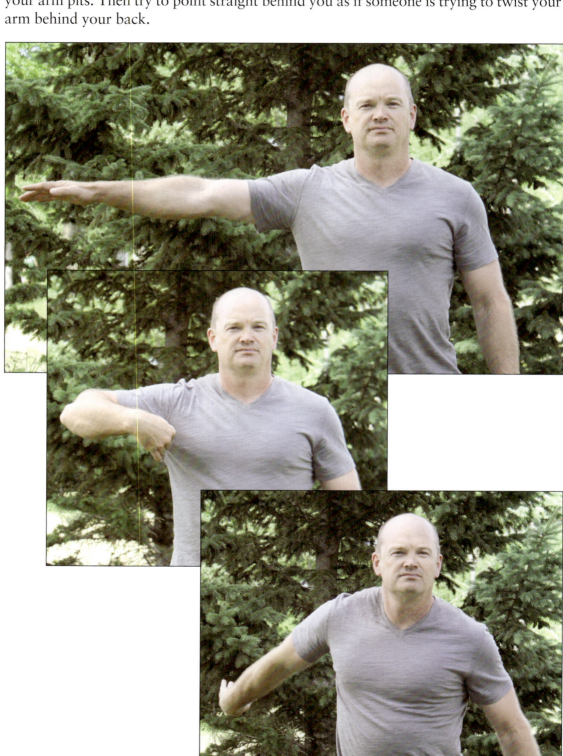

8. Puffed Chest and Sunken Chest

Inhale and stick your chest out. Now imagine someone has just punched you in the sternum. Exhale as you absorb the "punch".

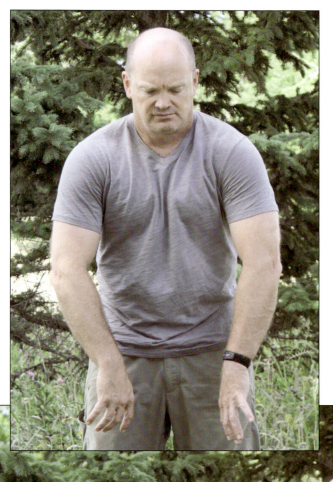
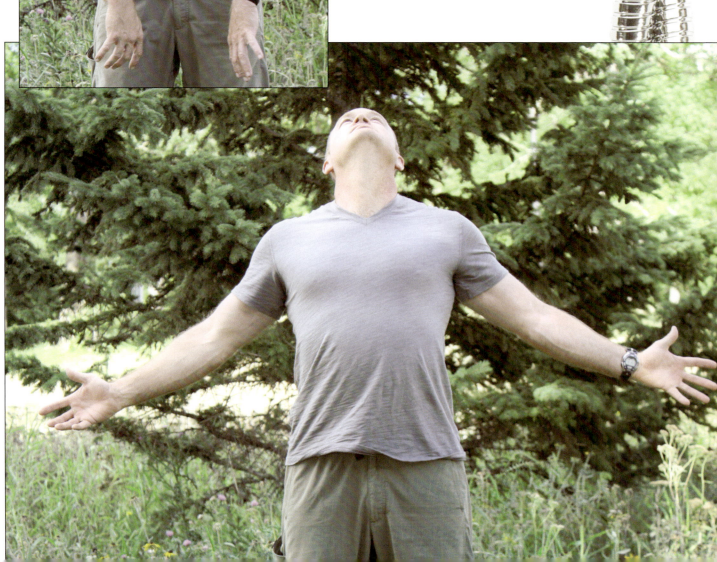

9. Shoulder Shrugs. (Both Shoulders Together)

Forward then backward. Keep the same in and out chest action going as in the previous drill, but combine that with some shoulder shrugs. Shoulders go up to your ears, then back as far as you can and finally down. Smooth the motion out. After you have completed the number of reps going backward, reverse and match them with the same amount of forward reps.

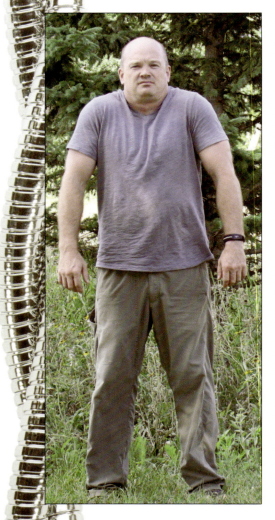
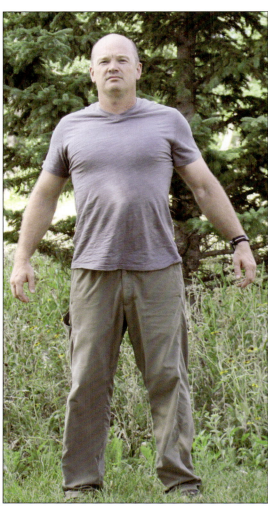
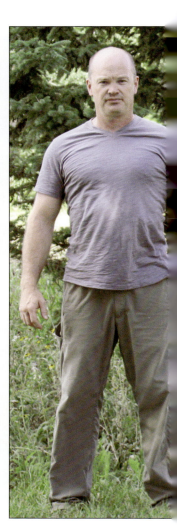

10. Shoulder Shrugs. (One at a Time) Forward and Backward

Same as previous just with one shoulder. Make sure both shoulders are moving and let the wave of motion go through your whole body.

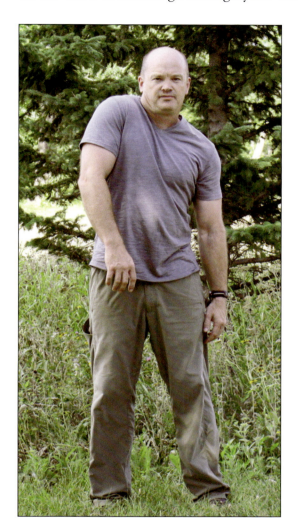
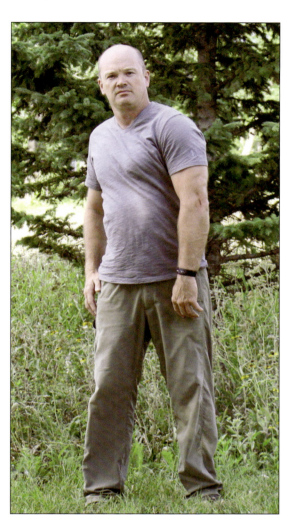

11. Pendulum Swings (Side to Side Similar to a Golf Swing)

Come up on the ball of one foot. Really strive to open up your hips.

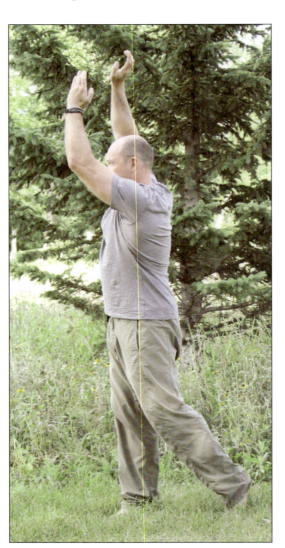
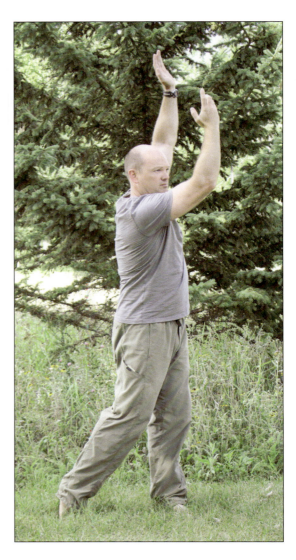

12. Elbows Locked Infinities (Horizontal Figure 8s)

Like rowing a kayak. Go both ways.

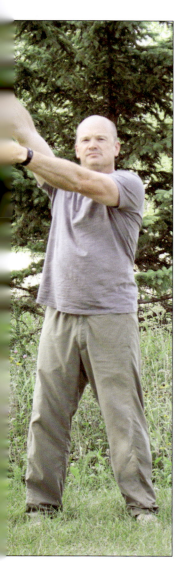
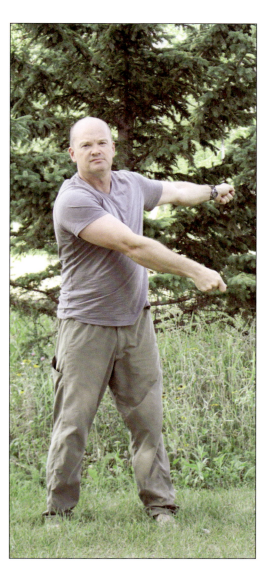
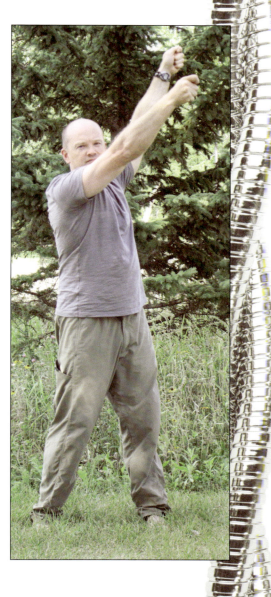

13. Vertical Figure 8 Arm Circles (Like a Rope Trick)

Go both ways.

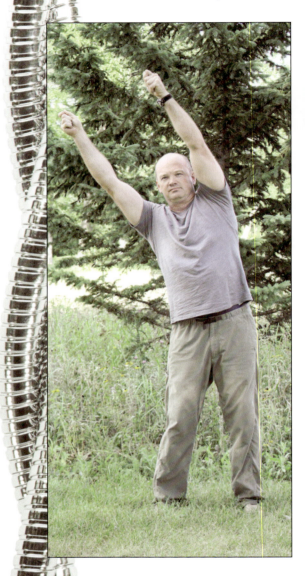
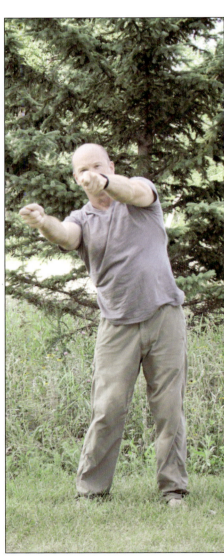
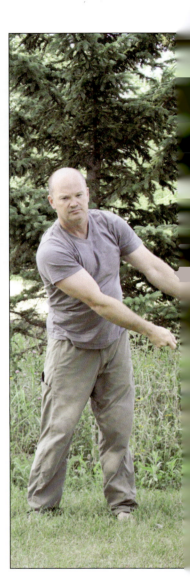

14. Arm Flings (Hug Yourself and Then Fling Your Arms Open)

Switch which arm goes on top every rep.

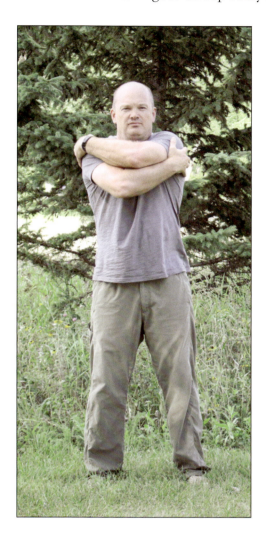 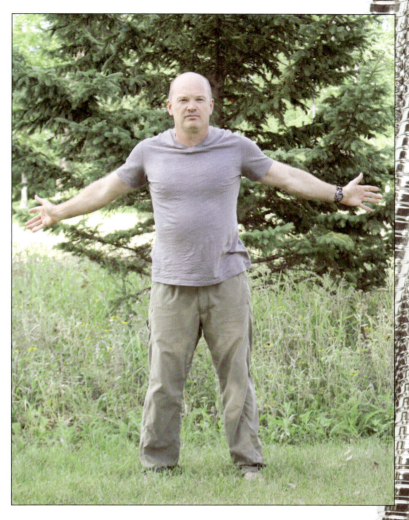

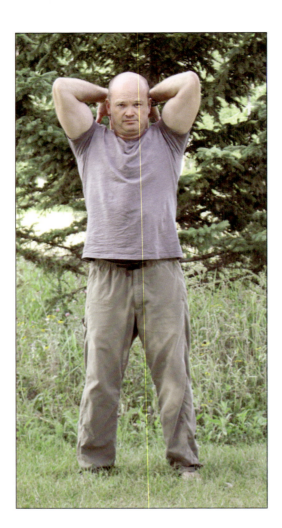

15. Tap Yourself on the Shoulders

16. Forward Arm Circles
Both arms together.

17. Backward Arm Circles
Both arms together.

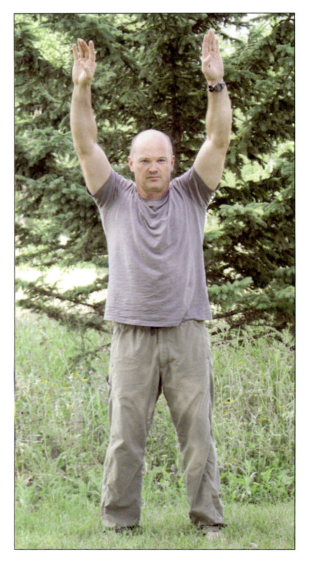

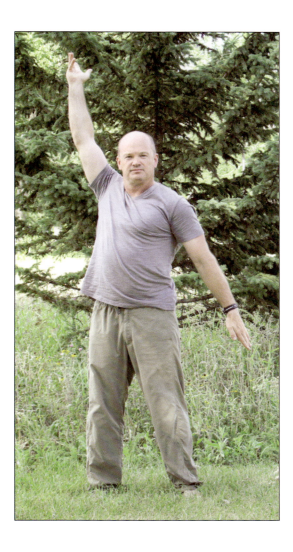

18. Single Arm Circles
Forward and then backward.

19. Alternating Arm Circles
Right arm goes forward—left goes backward and then switch.

20. Circle and Side Punch

Left arm circles forward as the right arm punches out to the side. Then switch.

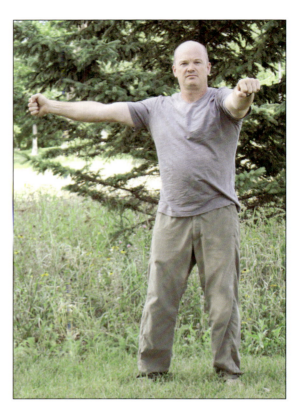

21. Twists with Taps

Move from your center line and just let centrifugal force whip your arms around. Tap yourself lightly in the back and side.

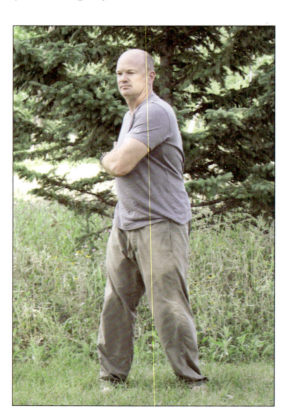
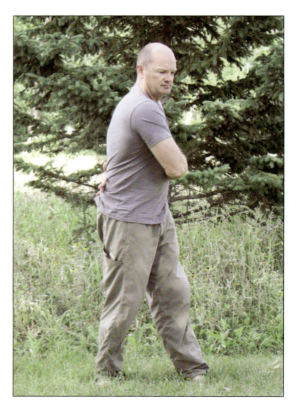

22. Side Bends

Imagine you are stuck between two plate glass windows, you must move strictly sideways.

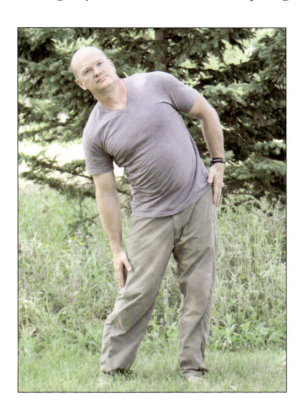

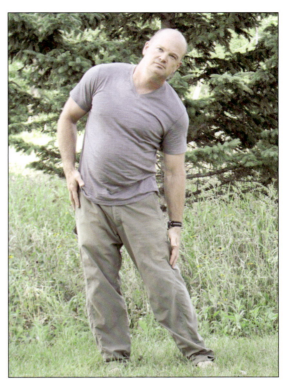

23. Pelvic Tilts

Make small forward and backward pelvic tilts, then side to side pelvic tilts like you are dancing a samba.

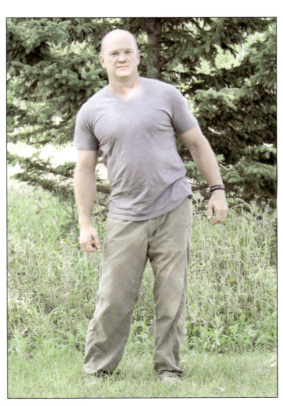

24. Belly Dance

Imagine you are standing inside a horizontal diamond. Touch each corner of the diamond with your hip. Smooth out the movement so it looks like a belly dance.

25. Hula Hoop Hip Circles

A more traditional hip circle from high school PE. Just make sure to slowly increase your range. Especially going to the back.

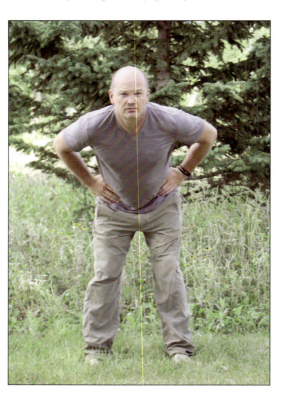
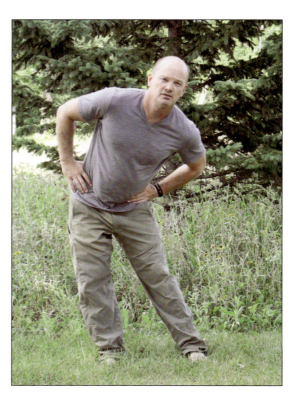
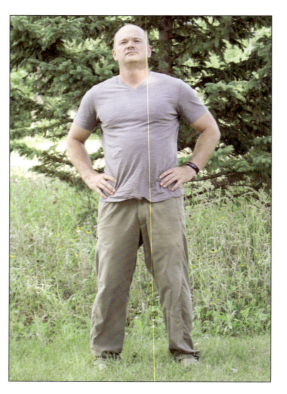
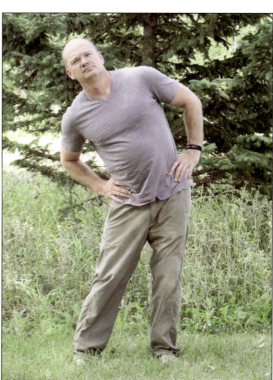

26. Leg Circles

Both directions. Make sure your knees stay locked and the movement comes from your hip.

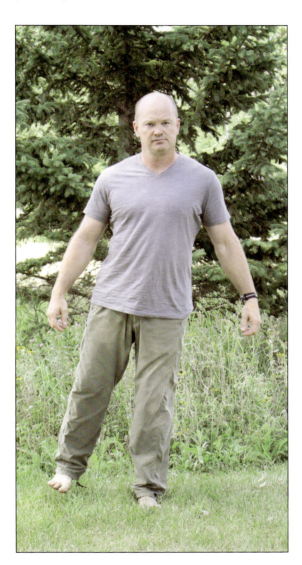
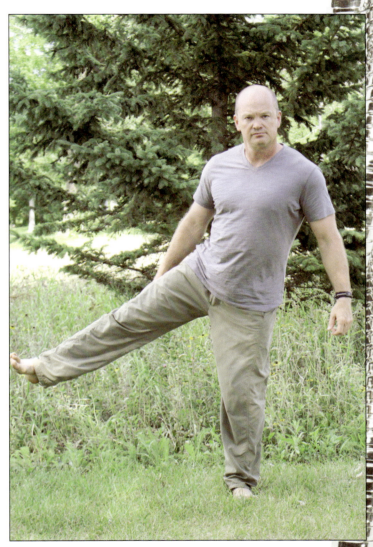

27. Knee Circles

Bring your knee up past belt level. Imagine your leg is dead from the knee down. Now make circles letting your lower leg dangle.

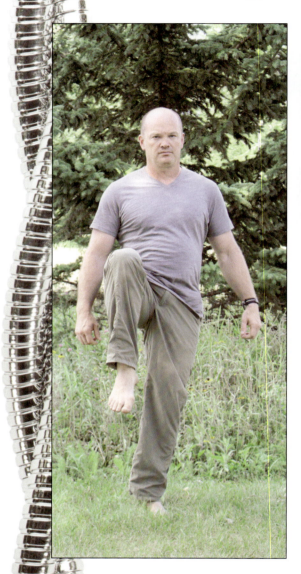
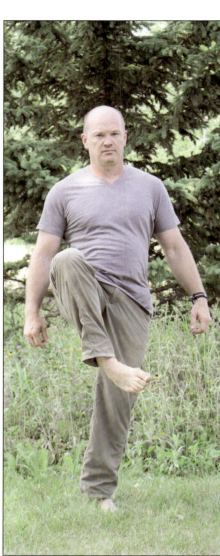
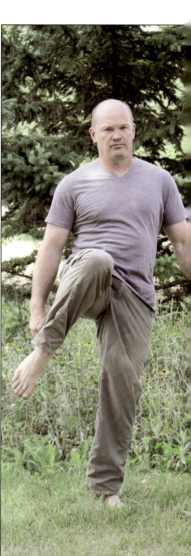

28. Standing Knee Circles

Closed chain. Keep both feet flat on the floor and make small knee circles. Make sure to lock out on top and don't look down at your feet.

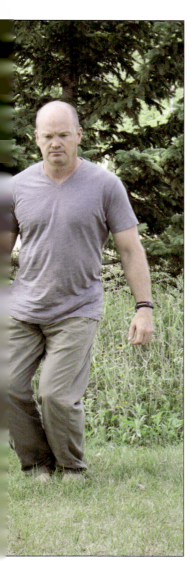
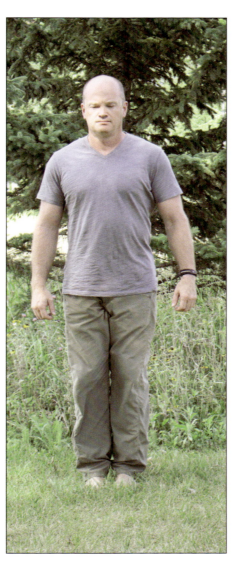
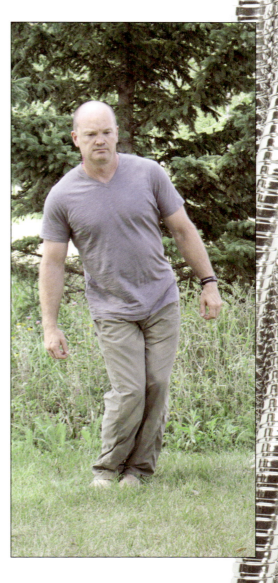

29. Ankle Circles

Just try to make smooth circles in both directions.

No ratchet movements.

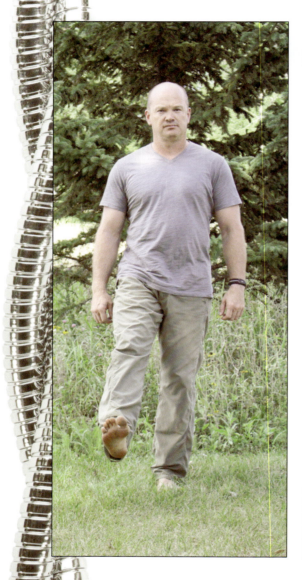
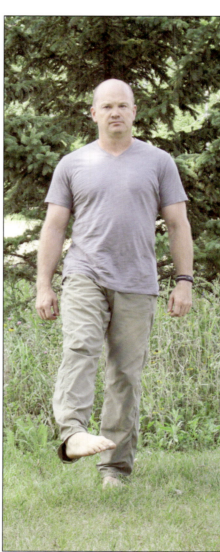
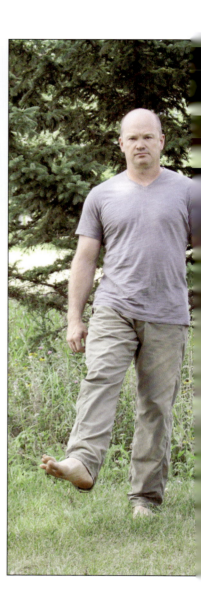

30. Bowing (Hip Hinges)

Make knife hands and push your hips back, keeping your weight on the heels. Knees should remain "soft". Chest big and back straight. Once you stand back up, contract your glutes, bend back and try to see the wall behind you.

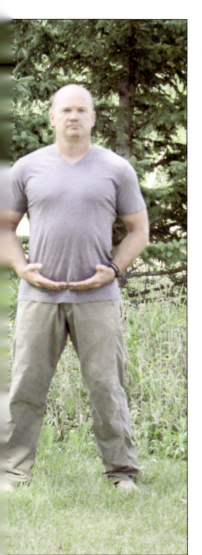
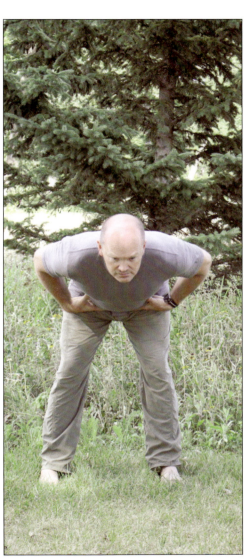
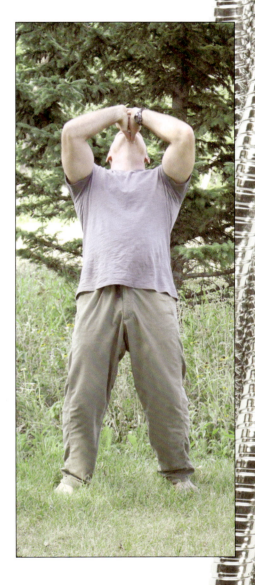

31. Squats

Make sure your knees stay in line with your index toe. Don't let your knees collapse inward or plié out. Imagine you are standing with your toes on a line. Don't let your knees or head drift over the line. Keep your back flat and chest big. Weight is on your heels. When you stand back up, tap your glutes to make sure you lock out between reps.

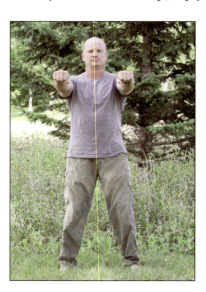 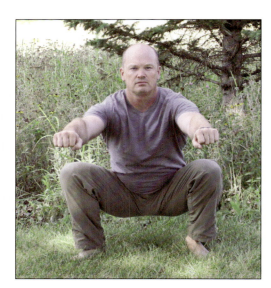

32. Side Lunges

Stand with your feet wider than shoulder width apart. Your feet should be pointed outward approximately 45 degrees. Squat on one leg keeping the other straight similar to a Kung Fu stance. Both feet stay in contact with the floor. Look at your straight leg. All the guidelines to squatting apply.

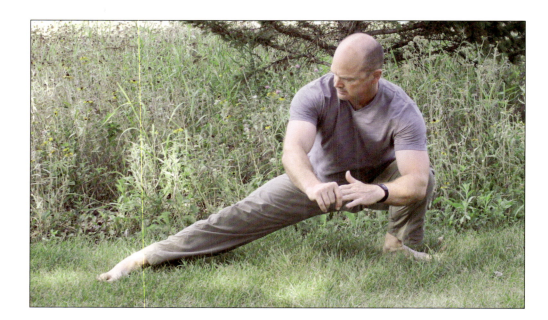

33. Cossack Switches

Start as above. Once you are down in the hole, turn your foot so your toes point to the sky. Make sure to keep the heel that you are sitting on down. You may use your elbow to "push" your hip open. Now imagine you are in a room with a very short ceiling. Switch sides by creeping into a horse riding stance and then go to your other side.

Stay low.

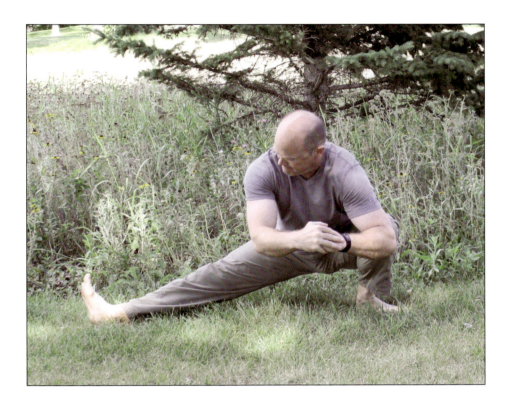

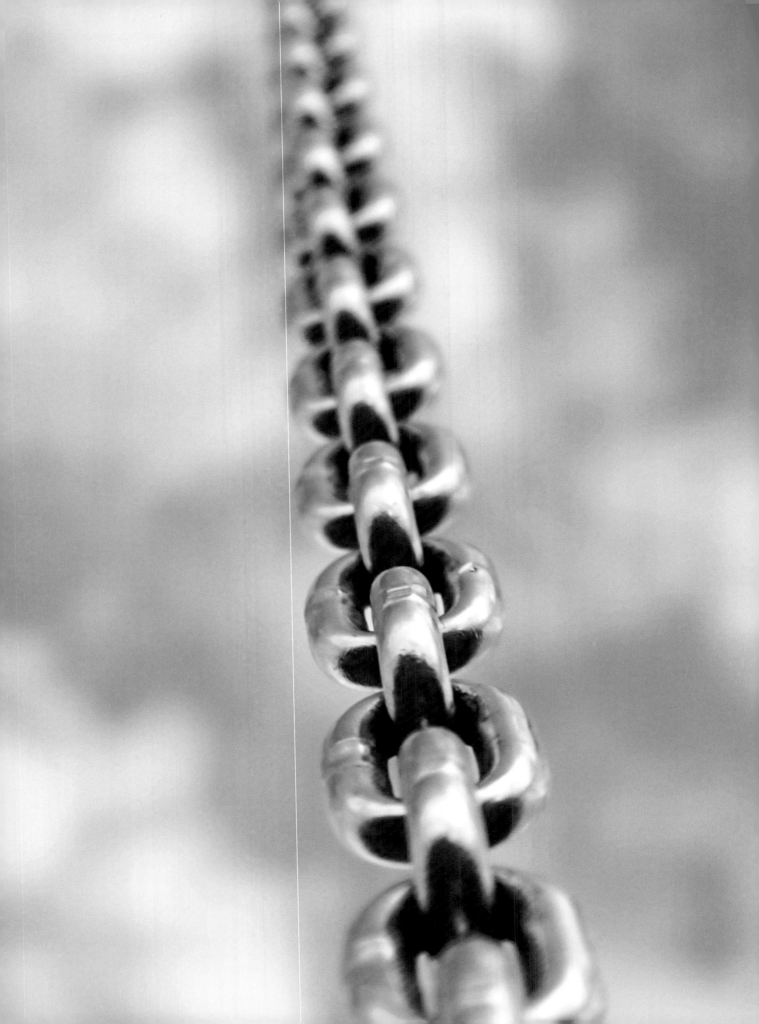

CHAPTER 6

Series 2: The Frog

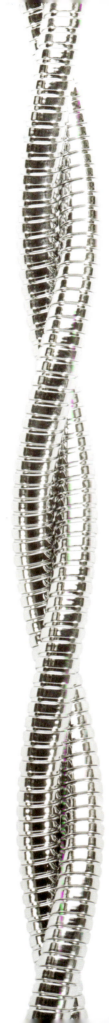

The Tactical Frog is a mobility/flexibility drill that will go a long way toward your quest for the side splits. If the side split is not high on your goal hit list, have no fear, you should still incorporate the frog sequence into your daily mobility training. If you are a martial artist, especially a kicker...this is a high return drill. Not a martial artist? The frog series will do amazing things for your ability to squat—and everyone should squat.

The frog is nothing new...martial artists and gymnasts hopefully have already been doing this, but what makes it special is the sequence that I use. This will optimize the effectiveness of your frog time.

The Pump

The pump is a great way to prepare your body for the rigors of the frog se ies. If you are familiar with yoga, the pump is an upward facing dog into a downward facing dog.

To perform the pump, get into a pushup position with your hands about shoulder width apart, fingers turned out at around a 45-degree angle. Your feet will be slightly wider than shoulder width. Keeping your elbows locked, push your hips in the air and extend your back. Try to push your heels to the ground. Look back between your feet and try to open up your chest. Make a few light, springy movements to further open up your chest. Keeping your arms straight, lower your hips and imagine you are wrapping your spine around a ball. Try to look at the wall behind you and do not let your feet collapse in. You have just completed 1 repetition. Do 10-20 repetitions. Finish in the up dog and let your knees touch the ground. Push yourself back and spread your knees to start stage 1.

Stage 1

Get down on the ground with the insides of your knees touching the mat. Make certain you have a nice soft, forgiving surface like a mat or—if you're lucky—outside in the soft grass works well. Turn or "frog" your feet out, well, like a frog. As for your arms, lock your elbows and brace yourself upright like you are doing pushups. Keep your back long and neutral and DO NOT let your spine flex. Be a little swaybacked rather than rounded...this is a frog not a turtle!

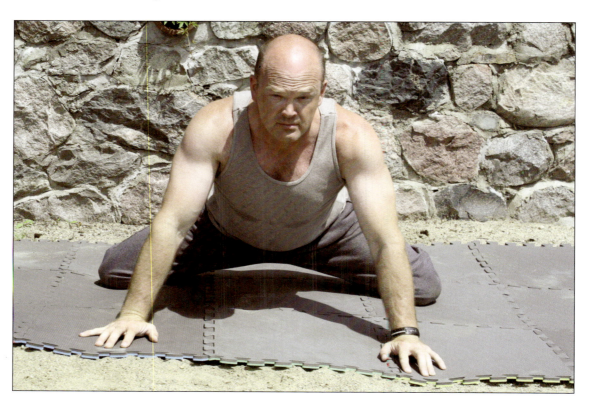

Slide your knees apart as if you are trying to do a side split. When you have spread your knees apart as far as they will go, begin slowly rocking back and forth. Go forward as far as you can and backward as far as you can go while maintaining spinal extension...tailbone must point to the sky. Repeat this rhythmical rocking for 10 to 20 repetitions.

Throughout this and all of the other stages try to spread your knees further and further apart and lengthen your spine.

Stage 2

During this stage keep your knees where they are and go down on your forearms. Continue your rhythmic rocking and try to lengthen everything. To explain this a bit more in-depth and for the sake of discussion imagine you are having an out-of-body experience and looking down on yourself from above. Your knees and head should form a triangle. What I want you to do is grow the points of your "triangle" longer. This visual will help you to find some extra space in your body allowing you to get your knees further apart and your groin closer to the ground. Repeat for 10 to 20 repetitions.

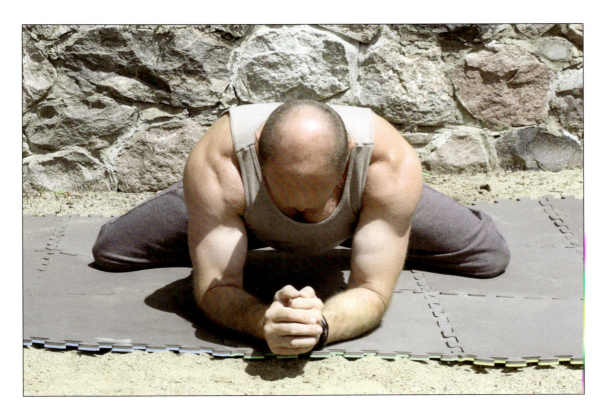

Stage 3

Keeping your hips back, and your elbows in the same place, rotate your right upper thigh as in a roundhouse kick, until the top of your thigh is on the ground and your right foot is by your right ear. Now switch and do the same thing on your left.

Repeat for 20 repetitions.

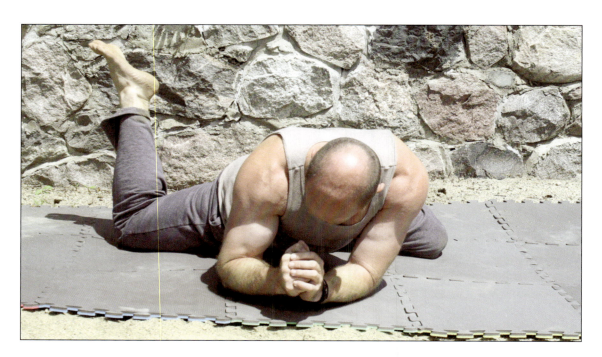

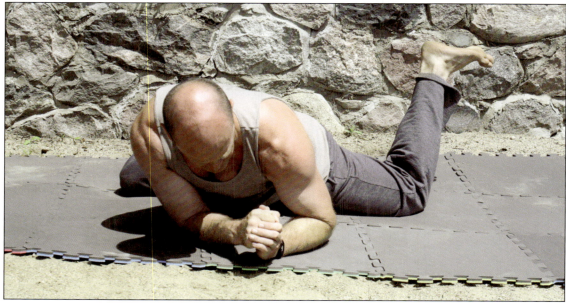

Stage 4

Go back and repeat stage 2 for another 10 to 20 repetitions. Your knees should spread apart even further.

You may choose to stop here if you are short of time or just starting out...if that is the case, take a short break and do the series 2 more times. If you have more time and want to fast track results read on.

Stage 5a

From the frog position straighten out your right leg. Lock your knee and keep it that way. The inside of your foot is on the ground, toes pointed forward and heel pointed back. Start rocking forward and backward as in stage 2, but this time you will have a straight right leg and a bent left leg. Lengthen and push away with your right heel and at the same time lengthen and push away in the other direction with your left knee. Keep moving and rocking the whole time. Repeat for 10 to 20 repetitions.

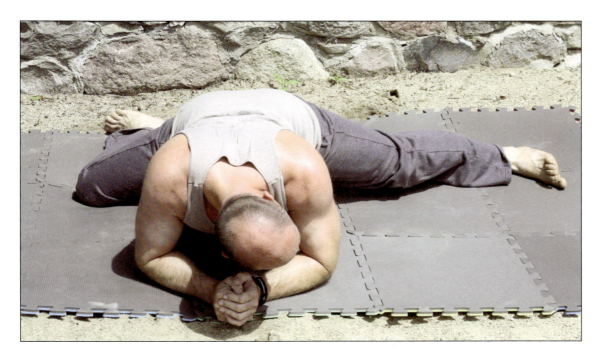

Stage 5b

From the above position, get upright by straightening your arms and rotating your hip...you should finish with the toes of your right foot pointing up at a 45-degree angle. This time when you are rocking you will also try to rotate from your hip, so when you go back your toes will point straight up at the sky and when you go forward your toes will be pointing forward... Foot parallel to the floor. Repeat for 10 to 20 repetitions.

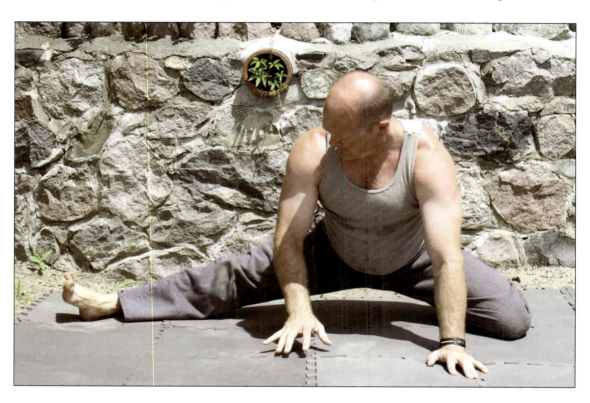

Stage 6

Re-bend your right knee and place it back on the ground, but try to put it down further away than it was. Straighten out your left leg and repeat stages 5a and 5b with your left.

Once you have completed the above stages you have a choice.
1. Stand up, shake the tension out of your body and start over. I recommend making 3 trips through.
2. Re-bend your left knee...place it further apart than when you started stage 6. Immediately go into another lap starting at stage 1. Again, try to go for 3 cycles if you have the time.
3. Continue on to stage 7a.

Stage 7a

From Stage 6 go down on your elbows again and straighten both legs, toes pointed forward, feet parallel to the mat. Move back and forth as in stage 5a. Really try to push your hips back with your elbows. Do 10 to 20 repetitions.

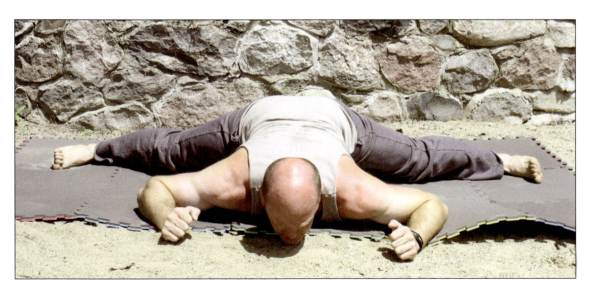

Stage 7b

Leaving your legs in a split position, get your body upright by straightening out your arms. Your toes will be pointing up to the sky because you have rotated from your hips. Begin doing split pushups. As you bend your arms to descend into the pushup let your hips roll so your toes are pointed forward. When you come up from the pushup let your hips roll so your toes are pointed to the sky. Keep in motion the whole time and try to push imaginary walls apart with your heels constantly.

Do 10 to 20 repetitions.

When you are finished, go into the low pushup position and bend your knees back into a frog. Now slowly crawl forward and bring your knees together. You may need a spatula to peel yourself off the floor.

Shake your hips out and do some squats to see the performance difference.

Note:

It is a good idea to chase the frog sequence down with a pigeon pose type stretch to relieve hip cramps.

Also, when you are doing the frog series it is important to relax and breathe deeply. Keep your face impassive. A screwed up face, shallow breathing and moaning and groaning like a 900 call center is a sure way to sabotage your results. Take your time and just slowly "melt" into the movements.

The tactical frog series is an essential lower body mobilizer that will make a huge difference in your kicks and squats.

Plug this into your training and drop me a line at info@extremetraining.net and let me know your results.

CHAPTER 7

Splits Defined

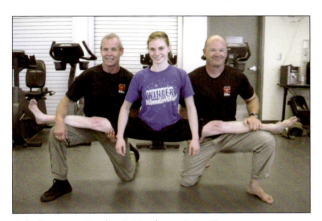

For the sake of discussion, clarification, and education, I should at this time define and describe the different species of splits. The splits can be classified into 3 basic species; each has its own specific benefits and uses.

Cole Summers, Stephanie Northway & Jon Engum

1. The Martial Arts Split

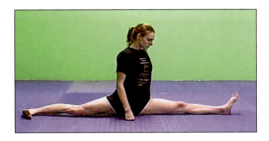

This split is the simplest and easiest to achieve and therefore I recommend it as the starting point of your split practice. The martial arts split is also very practical and beneficial to, you guessed it, the martial artist, as its form replicates many of the kicks performed in several different arts.

In the martial arts split, one foot is pointed toes up, as in a front kick, while the other foot is pointed sideways, as in a side kick. Face the front kick foot. The knees of both legs must remain locked throughout the exercise.

The martial arts split maybe used as a mobility drill to loosen up before attempting more aggressive splits, as in the hip switches described later on in the book, or as a standalone practice, read isometrics, to increase flexibility of the adductors and hamstrings and to a lesser extent the calf muscles.

2. The Front Splits

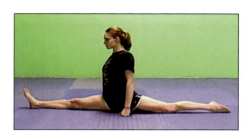

The front split—sometimes referred to as the gymnastic split—starts out similar to the martial arts split. The difference comes from the position of the back leg and foot. Instead of the back foot being sideways, it is pointed down to the ground; your instep is in contact with the ground as well as your back knee. Both your back foot and down knee of the same leg must form a straight line.

3. The Side Splits

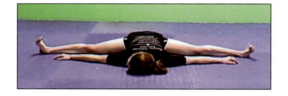

The side splits go by many different names, the Chinese Splits, the Dead Splits or the Russian Splits. Regardless the name you choose, the fact of the matter is that they are the hardest most challenging splits for the majority of people.

Perform the side splits by abducting your legs apart. Spread them sideways. Toes can be pointed up...targeting the hams. Pointed straight ahead targeting the abductors and groin muscles more, or at a happy medium around 45 degrees. Your back can be upright or you may choose to roll forward and lay your chest and elbow on the ground in front of you to perform what Pavel Tsatsouline calls the road kill splits.

See the chapter on stemming your way to the splits to help you conquer this leviathan of the splitting world.

Special thanks to Stephanie Northway, HKC for modeling the above splits.

Chapter 8

Stem Your Way to the Splits
Strategies for Eliminating Hip Pain from Your Splits

f you are on a journey into the splits, I have a few tips for you that will dramatically reduce the time and some of the agony of achieving your goals.

Note: this is especially important and effective for those who are feeling pain or discomfort in the top of their hips; the following techniques virtually eliminate this frustrating distraction.

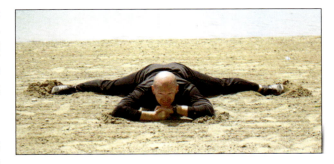

I happened upon these by accident while rock climbing. I was belaying my lovely wife and I noticed that she was able to perform some incredible acts of flexibility, that were way beyond her range when she was on terra firma.

What she was doing is called stemming in the climbing vernacular. Picture the old Western movie where the heroes are trapped at the bottom of a well. In order to climb out they get back to back and put their feet on the walls and use counter pressure to slowly walk up the well walls.

Climbers normally stem when they are negotiating a diphereal, a corner that is like an open book, and they put their right foot and right hand on the right wall and left foot and left hand on the left wall and use counter pressure to wedge themselves up the climb.

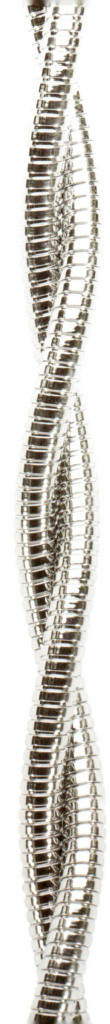

All is well and good until the walls start to open up and you find yourself getting stretched out into the side splits.

The interesting thing about this is that the climber is generally able to achieve a much greater and relatively pain free split than when they are on the ground.

Why? Is it because of the increased adrenaline that the body is putting out because you are dangling 50ft in the air?

Is it just reciprocal inhibition of the muscles working to wedge yourself onto the wall?

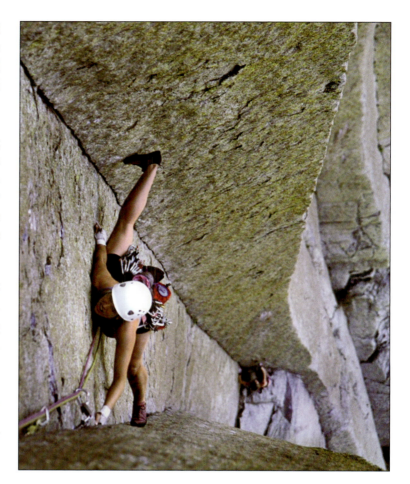

Is it the fact that you know there is no physical way that your feet can slip further out so you feel you are safe?

I have some theories, but the important thing is that it works—and I will show you a few ways to exploit this without having to take up climbing.

Fast forward a couple weeks and I am running in the Spring thaw. I decided to work some split switches as part of my mobility cool down.

A split switch is the martial arts split, front foot pointed up and back foot in a sideways or side kick position and then you switch so the opposite foot is pointed up. In the process of switching you need to travel through a side split position.

Anyway, the process of switching back and forth naturally digs holes in the soft Spring ground giving, you guessed it, walls. By pushing hard on these walls as if you are stemming you can get through the side split part without rising up, something that is normally done, hmmm. No pain. No pressure.

So next, I just stayed in the side splits and begun rocking forward and backward. Comfortably!

Aha! The effect has nothing to do with being high up in the air but all to do with the pressure of the stem.

So here is my plateau-busting, breakthrough method. Hopefully you will see the same amazing results that my students and I have.

Method 1—AKA Dig Your Own Hole

Go to the beach in the sand. Pavel has often recommended split practice in the sand. He says you can pile up the sand to relax on, or for the mutants dig sand out and practice negative splits. I will focus on the former because if you are doing negative splits you do not need my advice.

Start digging holes with your feet by the back and forth motion of split switches as described above.

Really focus on pushing the sand away from your center. When you have created sufficient "walls", hit your center splits and really wedge yourself in with counter pressure.

Now start working back and forth. Roll forward and then back. It should be fairly comfortable.

Next hit center and start performing contractions as if you are trying to slide your feet together. If you have not read Pavel's **Relax into Stretch**, stop and do so. That book covers the contract-relax part of this. You need this book. Goodbye comfort. Hello pain. The focus should now be on getting stronger, so hold your contraction as long as you can tolerate it.

When you cannot stand it any more, relax. Push very hard on the walls you have created and do some more prying and deep breathing.

Crawl safely out of the stretch and shake loose.

This is the first of 3 to 5 sets.

Each sequential set, "dig" your walls further and further apart.

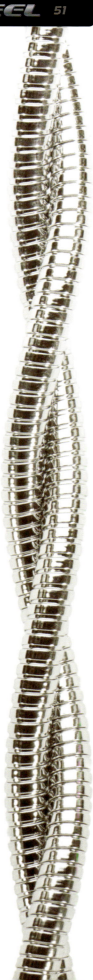

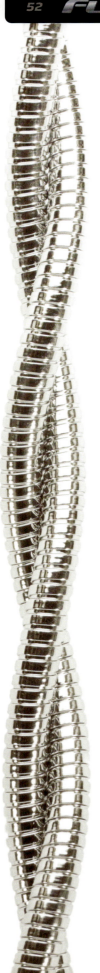

Advantage: This method gives you a very comfortable relax phase of the forced relaxation practice.

Disadvantage: You need to go to the beach and you have to restart the set to get lower.

Method 2—AKA It's In The Bag

Being a TKD instructor, I have access to several free standing heavy bags, the kind whose base is filled with water and weigh about 200 lbs.

Position two of these bags apart approximate to your splits and begin the hip switches as before. This time you are pushing your feet against the bags' base. When you are comfortable with that width, your partner can ever so carefully inch the bags apart.

Carry on as before.

Advantage: You can work in the gym and you do not need to come out of position to get wider.

Disadvantage: You need heavy bags and a partner.

Method 3—Bells Stand Alone

Place two heavy kettlebells, 40kg, on their sides, bottoms facing each other. Get in between them and begin the split switches. When you are as far as you can go, hit the side splits again and wedge yourself between the bells. After you have pried side to side and done some contractions, you may spread the bells by plantar-flexing your feet.

Advantage: You can do this anywhere. No partner is needed. You can adjust the width yourself in position, and it has the added benefit of you being able to measure exactly how far the bells are apart at the end of the training session. This will let you track your progress.

Method 4—AKA 3's Company

When I spoke to Pavel about this, he liked it but he put his own evil spin on it. "Jon perhaps you should have a couple of training partners let you push on their feet and then without warning take them away an inch or two and repeat."

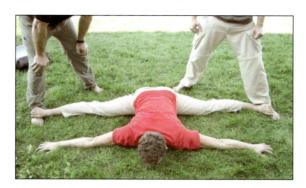

Truly wicked, but effective.

Ratcheting Mini Tensions

Here is one last advanced tip. When you get as far as you can with your regular contractions, try some mini-contractions. Just turn the power on and then quickly off. Do not do so explosively, just on and off and match the exhales with the off phase. Kind of ratchet your way down. This is an extreme power tool but it will get you flatter than road kill.

Try these out and see what works for you. Steve Freides, you know the guy who came back from a devastating back injury to achieve the suspended splits between chairs, gave me some advice sometime ago. "Mix up the surface that you split on. Sometimes use a slippery surface and other times use a sticky non-sliding surface." I will add to his sage advice. Put the above methods into your practice and be amazed.

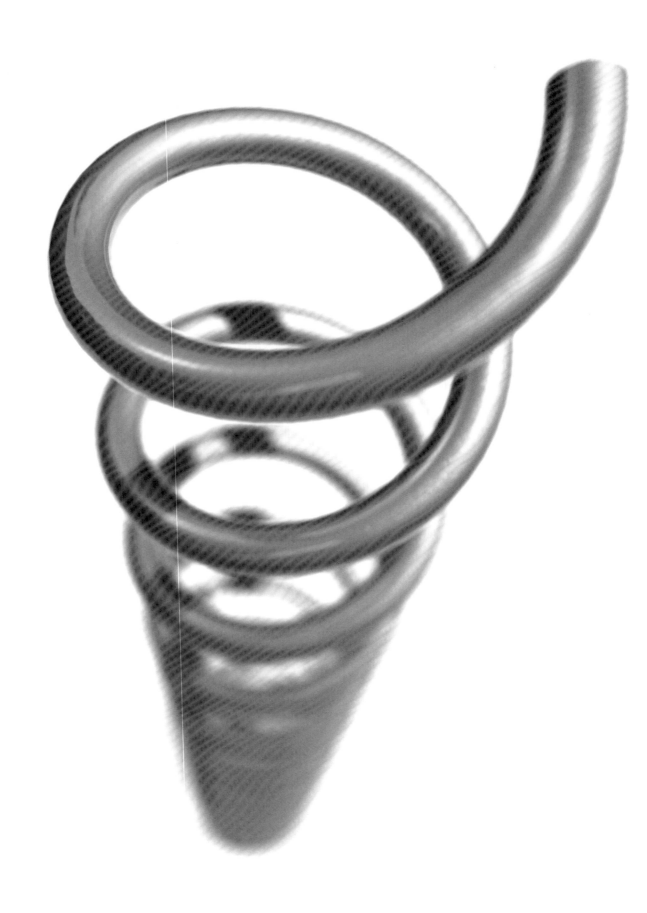

Chapter 9

Front Splits for Back Health

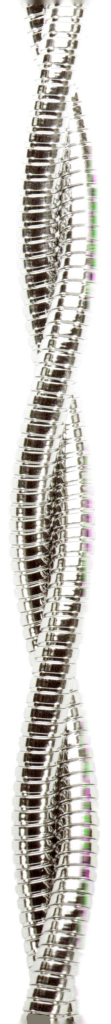

It has been said time and time again that one of the most common contributing factors leading the way to back pain is tight hamstrings and/or tight hip flexors.

Sure other things play a role as well, but Americans for one are plagued by lower back pain. This is no surprise since we are one of the heaviest and tightest groups of people on the planet.

We live in a "seated" culture, we sit to drive to work, we sit all day at work and then sit to commute back home, we sit to eat and to relax, and some sit to exercise. I am convinced this is the reason for the back problems many face and I offer the following story as proof.

I routinely teach seminars and workshops in Asia and during one of these workshops things were really put into prospective for me. I was teaching a group of around 30 personal trainers on the finer points of kettlebell training, and one of the subjects on the docket was how to front squat. Well I knew this was going to be a breeze when the group dropped into perfect squatting form to fill out the registration forms that morning. But I figured we should still cover the hows of teaching the front squat because they were most likely going to face clients not as limber as those present.

As we proceeded working our way through the squat progressions, low and behold I found one woman out of the 30 that could not squat. Now all of the attendees were Korean but only this one gal could not squat. Upon further investigation it turned out that my non-squatter had been adopted from Korea at a young age and led most of her life in the States. She had just recently moved back to Korea...although this is purely anecdotal it does drive home the fact that inherent flexibility is neither gender nor race dependent, but has everything to do with lifestyle and culture.

So...back to the States and our poor sore lower backs. More often than not many clients report immediate relief once they actually stretch the hams and hip flexors correctly. Of course, people need to clear this with their medical professionals, but overall simply releasing these tight overworked muscles will bring some measure of relief.

One of the gentler hip flexor stretches is the kneeling lunge stretch and this is where you should start if you are new to this work.

Kneeling Lunge Stretch

Get into a lunge position by kneeling down on your right knee. The instep of your right foot will also be on the ground. Make sure to align your knee and back foot so they fall on the same line. Your front foot will be on its own line and your left knee will be in the air. Make sure your left shin, in this case, is vertical and your knee is tracking your front foot. Do not let your knee get in front of your toes.

Keep your hips square. If you can imagine that you have headlights on the crests of your hips, just make sure they both shine straight ahead. Now put your hands behind your back and push your hips forward. You should feel a stretch in the area of your front thigh and hip, kind of where your front pocket is. Push into and back out of the stretch using a rhythmical movement. The tempo should be 1 second forward and 1 second backward.

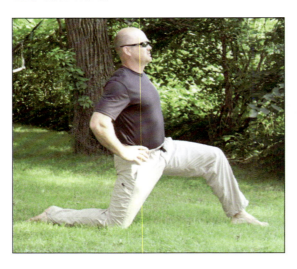 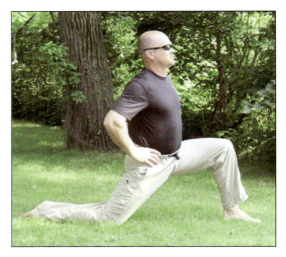

Quick Tips

- Contract the glute of the stretching side to a) protect your back and b) relax the hip flexors through reciprocal inhibition.

- If and when your knee begins to creep in front of your toes, simply re-position your front foot into a deeper lunge.

- Sigh when you are moving into the stretch and this will help relax the target muscles.

- Tilt your hips up, posterior tilt, before you even begin to stretch, to put the target muscles into a nice pre-stretch. This will further your efforts.

Good Morning Hamstring Stretch

The next weak link in the chain is the hamstring. One of the easiest and most effective stretches I know for the hamstrings is the good morning stretch and its several variations. Here is an extremely effective variant of the classic good morning.

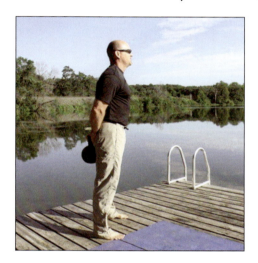
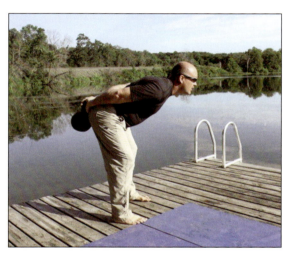

Quick Tips

- Stand completely upright, feet about shoulder width apart.

- Hold a kettlebell behind your back so that it rests more or less on your tailbone.
- Puff your chest out, big chest, and let your knees be "soft". It is not necessary or desirable to have them locked.

- Moving from your hips, try to push the kettlebell back with your tailbone while keeping your back straight and chest "big."

Do not worry about how far you bend over, this is not a toe touch. Just be concerned about how far back you can move the kettlebell. It is a hip hinge.

If you perform this move to the letter, you will feel a very intense stretch in the hamstrings just below your cheeks, not the ones on your face either ;).

Putting It All Together

Once you get proficient at the kneeling lunge stretch and the good morning Stretch you will want to move on to the Front Splits.

The front splits will give you two big bangs for one buck; you will be able to stretch the notorious hip flexors and hamstrings all in one shot. While the subject of this piece is front splits for back health, it should be noted that the front split will hyperextend the spine to a degree and may not be appropriate for everyone. Please clear this with your Doc. If you can handle it, the front split is a great time saving stretch for the above trouble makers.

Before you do front splits take a minute or two to stretch your calves—it will make for a much easier time once you do.

The RIF Calf Stretch

The following is a calf stretch from Master RKC Mark Reifkind.

- Stand facing a wall.

- Put the front of your foot on the wall in such a way that the toes are bent back and the ball of your foot is in contact with the wall.

- The rest of your foot should make a 45 degree angle from the ball of your foot to the heel. The heel is resting on the floor.

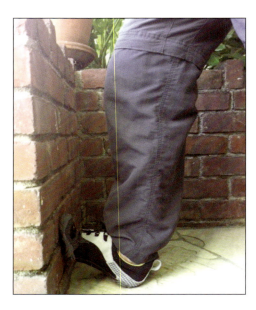 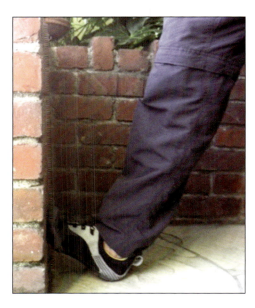

- Now simply push your hip forward toward the wall until you feel a nice stretch in your calf.

- Play around with the angle of your foot and the bend of your knee in order to hit the different muscles in your calf.

You are now ready to begin the front splits.

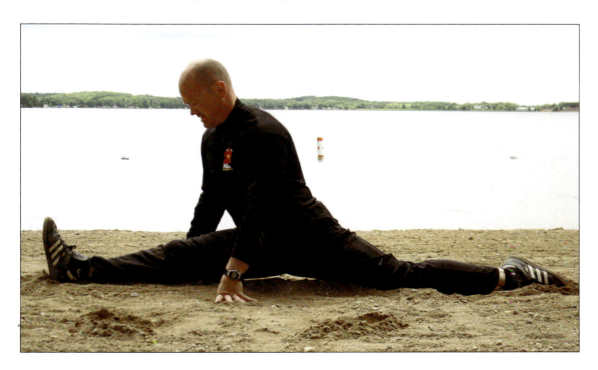

To get the best results you will need some kind of slippery surface to work on. I recommend getting some furniture movers. Furniture movers are small plastic discs that you can put under the legs of heavy furniture that allow you to easily slide your couch or other heavy things around the living room. Many of them have a slippery hard surface on one side and a padded surface on the other. They will also allow you to slide effortlessly into a deeper split. You can find them at any home supply store.

Set yourself up between two kitchen chairs for balance. Put your back knee on one of the furniture movers and the instep of your back foot on another. Your front heel will go on yet another furniture disc. Begin by doing the kneeling lunge stretch and when you feel up to it, push your right or front leg forward and straight ahead—at the same time push your back foot back.

Quick Tips

- Use contract-relax stretching in reps and sets, think 3 to 5 reps or contractions for 3 to 5 sets.

- Combine the contract-relax with gentle rocking from side to side—perpendicular to the direction you are trying to go. Example: contract or tighten up all your muscles and then relax with a sigh, immediately go deeper into the stretch and begin rocking and prying side to side.

- Every once in a while wiggle your front foot back and forth (plantar-flex and dorsi-flex) in an effort to relax and gain a few more centimeters of stretch.

Plug in the front splits to your health routine.

CHAPTER 10

Just Add Water

*"Mother, mother ocean I have heard your call...
in your belly you hold the treasure
few have ever seen . . ."*
—Jimmy Buffet *A Pirate Looks at 40*

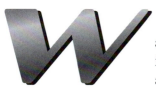ater is the giver of life. The sustainer of the earth, the primordial fluid our ancestors first crawled out of. The human being has always had a connection or a call to the water.

Want to ease your way into a greater range of movement? I suggest taking your training into the water. Now I am not talking about joining the local water aerobics class and prancing around in a Speedo to the golden oldies, not that there is anything wrong with that. Whatever floats your boat. Nor am I suggesting joining some cult and having a new aged, spiritual communion with the water lilies during a full moon. No talking to plants here my friend. I have a much more pragmatic approach. Read on.

We have already established the fact that to increase a stretch we must increase the muscles' ability to relax and display their full length. The problem is that to do any kind of split or extreme end range movement, you have to be somewhat proficient at the move to even begin to get into the correct starting position. This can be problematic for several reasons. If your muscles are already fighting you at the get-go, you are going to have a long uphill battle to improve. Perhaps you are a little stiff from training....this will also prevent or at the very least make it harder and more painful to put the relaxed stretching idea into practice. One solution is to go to the water.

Most modern yoga classes use props and bolsters to help their newbies get into a yogic posture, or asana, that may be beyond their current ability.

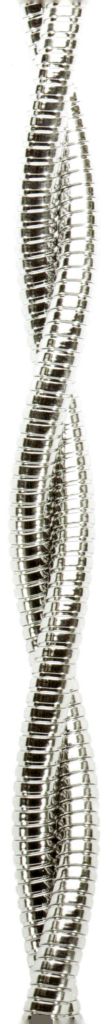

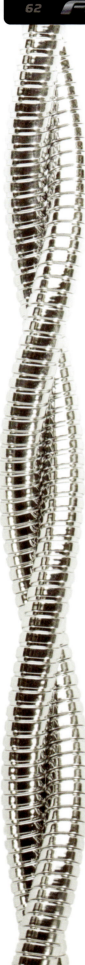

The purpose is twofold.

The bolster or cushion will take some if not all the weight off of the limb so the muscles can relax and get the student into a perfect alignment.

The yogi instructs the student to then relax, breathe deep and attempt to *melt* into the stretch...as the student becomes more pliable, the bolster or prop is lessened and gradually over time eliminated from the posture.

So to sum it up...support can be beautiful.

The other reason is to instill confidence and make the practitioner feel safe. If you do not feel safe during a stretching session there is little chance that you will be able to relax.

All of the above is well and good but I want to introduce you to a better mouse trap.

Specifically, the Beach

Go to the beach and use the water as your bolster. Let me explain.

You need to do a little searching to find the perfect location....but the search will be well worth it. What you are looking for is a warm body of water with a nice, gradually sloping, sandy bottom. You are looking for stretching nirvana.

It goes without saying that you want to avoid water that is infested with nasty sea creatures...no sharks, jellyfish, sharp coral, leaches and the like. If you do choose to practice in a place that has these dangers, then it will just be an act of natural selection and the gene pool will be better off. Say thank you.

Seriously, here is what you do.

The water depth in which you will start will depend on where you are at in your journey toward the splits. If you are a beginner, start out in water that is around waist deep. For more advanced people just a couple of inches will do. The shallower the water, the harder this will be. When in doubt, start deep.

Face toward shore so you will be looking "uphill".

Begin by practicing the kneeling lunge stretch. You may slowly "tread" water with your hands (think lazy breast strokes) to move you in and out of the stretch.

If you have gentle surf, that can work just as well. No crashing waves.

When you feel ready, push your lead leg forward into a front split. Now you may really focus on relaxing and gradually "sinking" into the stretch. The water will support most of your weight and you will find that it is very easy to move into a split. Gently rock side to side and as you relax push your feet into a greater stretch.

You can and should hold the stretch for a looooonnng time. Combine deep breathing and gentle flowing motion of the water to lull you into a deeper stretch.

When you feel you can, move into shallower water. This will allow you to control exactly the amount of weight you put on the stretch; i.e. the more of your body that is out of the water the less buoyant you will be. The shallower the water the more weight the stretching muscles will have to bear.

Next practice the side splits in the same fashion.

Start in a little bit deeper water and slowly sink into the side split. Use your hands again to tread back and forth. Go from a toes pointing up split to a toes pointing forward split.

Every so often roll your hips and switch to a martial arts split...do these so called "hip switches" and then plant yourself into a wider version of the side split. When you cannot get any deeper into your split without your head going under water it's time to move into shallower water.

You have a couple choices when it comes to moving in.

Option 1: Simply stand up—move in and start another set from scratch.

Option 2: Leave your legs in a split and use your arms to swim forward to the shallows.

Spend some time at this practice and be patient.

It is relaxed stretching after all.

Combine this water training with some deep meditative breathing and you will have a great recovery program.

- Training in the water like this will allow you to keep your back and the rest of your body in perfect position, even if you are not quite there on land.

- It will also allow you to manipulate how much tension you feel by either increasing or decreasing your buoyancy.

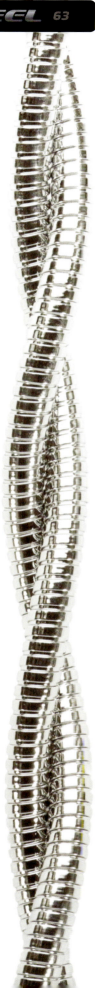

- It will increase your ability to relax in these extreme positions; why else would people buy wave machines to listen to the sound of the ocean?

Use the water training as just another arrow in your stretching quiver, but not as an end-all strategy.

Like our ancestors, you cannot stay in the water forever. Once you evolve you will need to wiggle your way toward shore and become a land animal.

A very flexible land animal at that!

CHAPTER 11

Escape Your Fighting Stance

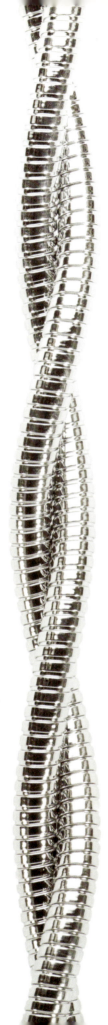

Do you live in the stance of your particular sport? Whatever your sport may be, are you guilty of living in that stance or position 24-7? Is that a healthy posture for you to be in? I first heard it put into words by Master RKC, Mark Reifkind who said "Do not live in the posture of your sport". I believe we are all guilty of it to some degree.

Let's face it, for a combat athlete, extension is a bad place to be. Most likely the only time you would be in extension during a fight is if you are down for the count. The typical fighter's stance is all about flexion, body crouched ready to spring, chin tucked in and shoulders hunched to protect the knockout button, a.k.a. the chin.

Okay so maybe you are not a combat athlete, but does the position described above differ much from the writer hunched over his computer or the truck driver at the wheel of his big rig?

For the most part, everyone lives in this posture and it is not a healthy place to be. To drive this point home take a field trip to any nursing home in the USA. Observe the way people are stuck in this posture shuffling around fighting themselves on each and every movement.

Pay particular attention to the frail old man who is nearing the end of his days hunched over and fighting gravity just trying to breathe. This is a fate we all face unless we take measures to counteract this deterioration.

The following mobility program will go a long way towards straightening you up.

First Analyze Your Posture

Stand straight, feet together and eyes closed. Start at your feet and work your way up to your head noting how you feel when you are standing at ease. Also notice how you feel in relation to the earth. Memorize this and we will come back to it after you complete the "Escape Your Fighting Stance" series.

Program Overview

The "Escape Your Fighting Stance" program features 3 exercise pairs done as supersets. Each subsequent set is taken deeper then the preceding set. After, and only after, you have completed 3 trips through the first pairings are you allowed to move on to the second group of exercises.

Superset 1

Rib Pull or Brettzels
Supersetted with RKC Armbars
3 X 8-10

Superset 2

Pumps or Hindu Pushups
Supersetted with Tactical Frogs
3X 8-10

Superset 3

Goblet Squats
Supersetted with Lunge stretches

Execution

Rib Pulls OR Brettzel

The rib pull or Brettzel was systematized and coined by the **Functional Movement System** guru Gray Cook and named after Master RKC, Brett Jones. Check out http://www.fms.com for more information on the blueprint for better movement.

Start both exercises the same way, lying completely on your side, shoulders stacked one on top of the other and some type of cushion under your head so that it remains straight and relaxed. For the sake of discussion we will assume you are lying with your right side on the ground. Next, bend your left knee and slide it up until it is above your belt line…the top of your left leg must at least form a 90 degree angle from your body. This angle will ensure that the movement comes from your thoracic spine and not the lumbar vertebrae. Pin the left knee to the ground using your right hand to hold down the top of your left leg. Now try to grow the line formed by your right leg, back, and neck. In other words, get your right heel and the top of your head as far apart as possible. Congratulations, you are now in the starting point of both the Rib Pull and the Brettzel.

The Rib Pull

To do the Rib Pull, and I recommend you start with it, reach across your body with your left hand and grab the right lower ribs to encourage the movement to come from the T-spine. Rotate to your left by pulling on your ribs. Rotate everything, head, neck, and ribs while keeping your right knee in contact with the ground. Once you get as far as you comfortably can, take some deep, relaxing belly breaths. Try to "melt" further and further into the movement. Do not forget about the 3 big S's that we talked about 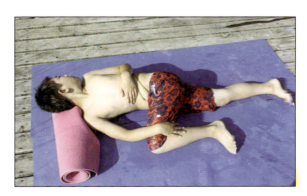 earlier. Work slowly and consistently to get your left shoulder to the deck while keeping your left knee in contact with the ground. Don't cheat the movement to get this or you will miss to whole point of the drill. Once you have had enough, slowly come out of the rotation and do your other side.

The Brettzel

Begin by assuming the starting position described above with one small addition. Bend your right leg by flexing your knee and grab your right instep with your left hand. Keep your hips fully extended and feel a stretch in your right thigh and hip flexors. The rest of the exercise is the same as above.

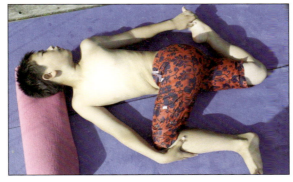

On both the Rib Pull and the Brettzel, feel free to move rhythmically into and out of the stretch. One move in and one move out counts as one repetition.

The RKC Arm Bar

The Arm Bar may be one of the most powerful, life-changing movements in the RKC arsenal. The effect of the arm bar on the shoulders, T-spine and all around posture is apparent as soon as you perform the movement. You can instantly feel a dramatic improvement and an opening throughout your entire body.

Let's examine the classic arm bar technique. The RKC arm bar starts out the same as its more familiar cousin the Turkish getup. I write this assuming you already know how to do the getup. If you do not know the getup then stop reading now and get thee to an RKC Instructor and learn the getup.

Lie on the floor with a light kettlebell on your right side. Grab the kettlebell with a pistol grip, right hand on the inside and left on the outside, pull your elbow to your ribs then roll on to your back prying the kettlebell up as you go. Now using both arms press the bell into the firing range position just as you would for the getup. Things start to differ from the getup at this point. Your left arm goes over your head (horizontally) while you are keeping the kettlebell or "working" arm perpendicular to the ground (vertically.) To quote Pavel Tsatsouline from the HKC manual, *"Using your left arm and leg as the axis of rotation and leaving the right arm with the kettlebell straight and vertical, bring your right knee towards your chest and roll to your left. Straighten out your right leg and lay it on the ground. Your feet should be a shoulder's width apart or wider, your knees straight, your toes pointed."*

At this point in the movement you will have 4 primary things to focus on.

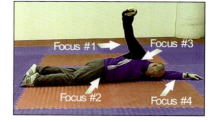

Focus #1
The kettlebell and working arm must maintain vertical (keep the kettlebell arm vertical in all planes without actually looking at the bell.) Rest your head on the left arm.

Focus #2
Rhythmically begin pumping your hips, trying to get the right hip, in this example, to the ground. It will help to contract the right glute, and breathe, sighing into the extension. The timing should be one rep every two seconds.

Focus #3
Try to make your right collar bone or chest area longer.

Focus #4
Wiggle the left arm (the one on the ground) further and further behind you. Think of stretching the lat.

When you have had enough *sloooowly* reverse the above process under full control.

Pumps or Hindu Pushups

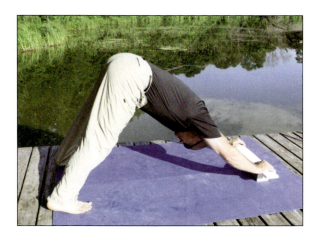

Tactical Frog

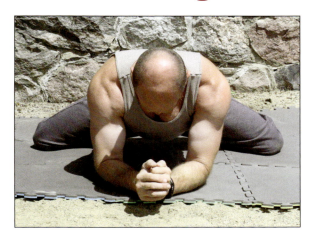

A quick tip on grouping #2.

You can flow seamlessly from the pump to the frog by doing the following:

When you have finished the required reps of the pump or Hindu pushup, end in the "up dog" position. Now let your knees touch the ground and push yourself back, opening your knees to the tactical frog start position.

Goblet Squats

Grab a kettlebell by the handle, kind of like grabbing onto a steering wheel. Pavel calls this "taking the bell by the horns." Squat down by sitting back and down between your heels.

The following goes without saying, but I will say it anyway:

- Make sure your knees line up and stay lined up with your toes. Your knees must point the exact same way your toes do through the whole squat.

- Keep your heels on the ground and your shins vertical.

- Keep your back straight, do not allow your tailbone to tuck under at the bottom of the squat.

- Keep a "big" chest, especially at the bottom.

- At the bottom, place your elbows to the insides of your knees without losing the alignment of your back. Use your elbows to push the knees out to help open your hips. Your feet must stay firmly fixed to the ground.

- Make sure when you ascend that your hips and shoulders come up at the same time. Do not lead or "hitch" with your hips.

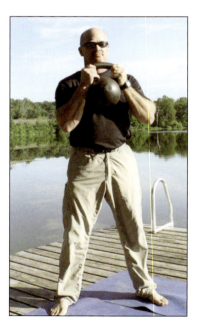
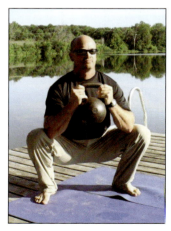
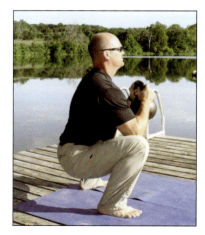

Lunge Stretch

Upon completion of the "Escape" program stand up and take a moment to re-assess your body. You should feel like a new person, taller, more upright, and downright free.

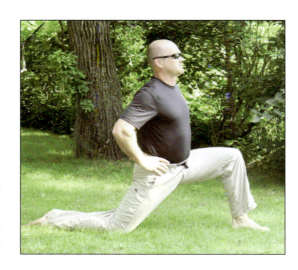

Practice this routine first thing in the morning as a recharge. Do it 3 times a week and give it at least a month. With dedicated and consistent practice you will turn back the hands of time.

I Challenge You!

Do not be a slave of your "sport."

Do not be satisfied with bad posture.

Break free from the crippling chains of time.

ESCAPE!

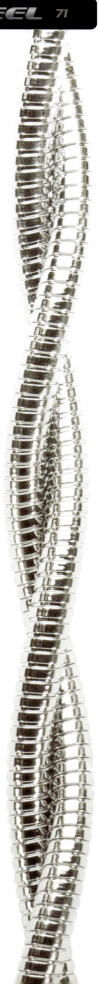

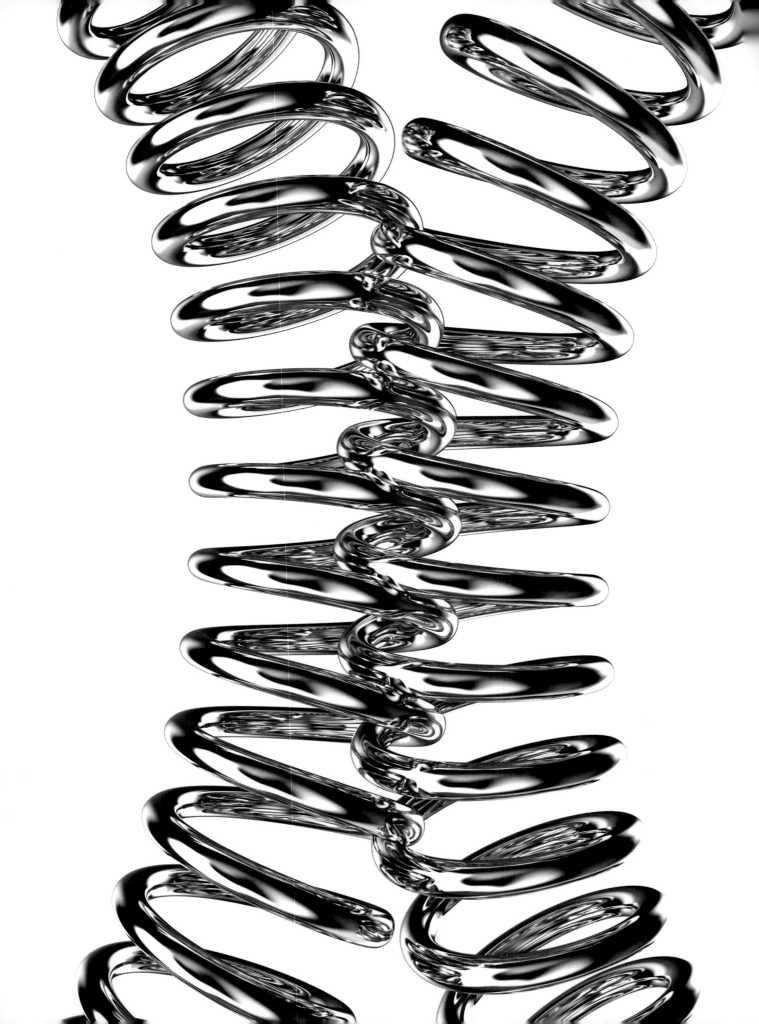

Resources

Dragon Door. http://www.dragondoor.com

Engum, Jon. Extreme Training http://www.extremetraining.net

Cook, Gray. Functional Movement System http://www.functionalmovement.com/

Tsatsouline, Pavel. *"Beyond Stretching"* DVD. St Paul: Dragon Door Publications, Inc., 2007

Tsatsouline, Pavel. *"Relax Into Stretch"*. St Paul: Dragon Door Publications, Inc., 2002

Tsatsouline, Pavel. *"Super Joints"*. St Paul: Dragon Door Publications, Inc., 2001

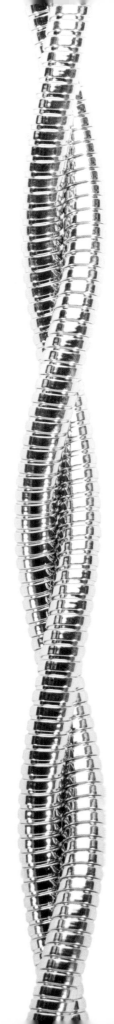

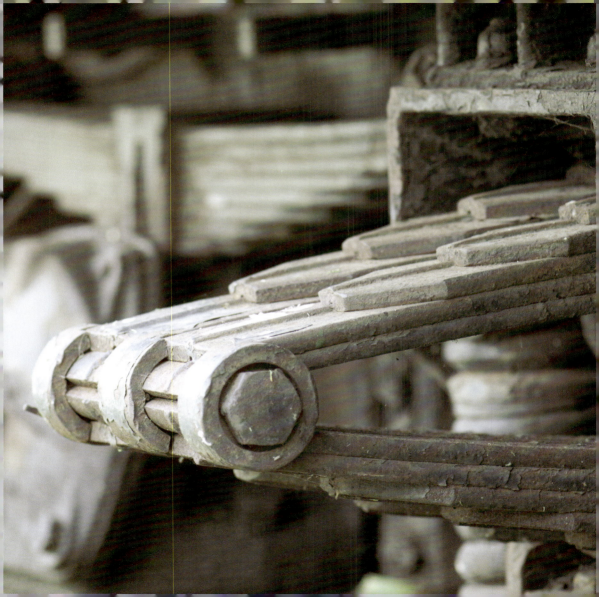

About the Author

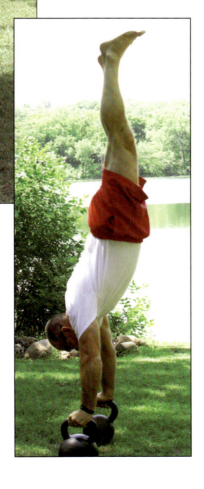

Jon Engum, Master RKC, CK-FMS. Holds a 7th Degree Blackbelt in Taekwondo, 4th Degree Blackbelt in Hapkido and 4th Degree Blackbelt in Kumdo. Grandmaster Engum is currently the #1 ranked RKC Instructor on the Dragon Door RKC page. He teaches Kettlebell, Flexibility, and Martial Arts Seminars World wide and can be contacted at *info@extremetraining.net*.

Praise for *Super Joints*

"The Do-It-Now, Fast-Start, Get-Up-and-Go, Jump-into-Action Bible for HIGH PERFORMANCE and LONGER LIFE"

Super Joints

"*Super Joints* by Pavel Tsatsouline was excellent. After 30 years of practicing and teaching martial arts (Uechi/Shohei Ryu, and Ju Jitsu), and the natural 'break down' of the joints with age, it has helped to restore the flexibility and strength of my joints, especially an arthritic shoulder."
—**Dr. Dan Rinchuse,** DMD, MS, MDS, PhD, Greensburg, PA, 6th Degree Black Belt Uechi/Shohei Ryu, 2nd Degree Black Belt Ju Jitsu

Easy to use with Powerful results!

"As a chiropractor and martial art instructor, I began incorporating the simple exercises with my patients and students. Everyone loves them. They get great results and are easy to do."
—**Donald Berry, D.C.,** Frederick MD

Joints of a teen again...

"At 37 years of age, my joints had already been cracking and hurting in the morning. I sustained an injury parachuting in the Air Force in 1989 and since, have had many back pains. I ordered *Super Joints* figuring it would be good, as all of Pavel's DVDs and books have been excellent. The first day I went through the DVD and did all the joint mobility drills. I felt better that day and over the course of the following week noticed that in the morning, my back wasn't as stiff and my elbows didn't hurt. I would highly recommend this DVD to anyone that cares about their joints."
—**Jim Lavelle,** NY

Back Pain Relief at Last

"I really enjoyed the *Super Joints* DVD. I have suffered from chronic low back pain for years without relief. Putting exercises into my daily routine has dramatically reduced my back pain and provided some long overdue relief from constant pain."
—**Mark Harrell,** Los Gatos, CA

DON'T BE A FOOL

"There are two reasons for not doing *Super Joints*. #1 you don't know about it. #2 You are a damn FOOL. I'm 49 and have had knee trouble all my life. I have done those big squats in my 20's and 30's (500lb+). I gave up squatting 39 and for the last 9 years I suffered with aching knees and was afraid to squat. I have been doing *Super Joints* for the last 6 months (have not missed a day). No more pain, no discomfort. This is my second copy. I love the way it makes my joints feel. Thanks, Pavel."
—**Scott G.,** Cedar Point, NC

Discover:

- The twenty-eight most valuable drills for youthful joints and a stronger stretch
- How to save your joints and prevent or reduce arthritis
- The one-stop care-shop for your inner Tin Man—how to give your nervous system a tune up, your joints a lube-job and your energy a recharge
- What it takes to go from cruise control to full throttle: The One Thousand Moves Morning Recharge—Amosov's "bigger bang" calisthenics complex for achieving heaven-on earth in 25 minutes
- How to make your body feel better than you can remember—active flexibility fosporting prowess and fewer injuries
- The amazing Pink Panther technique that may add a couple of feet to your stretch the first time you do it

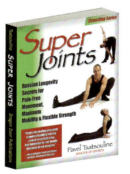

Super Joints
Russian Longevity Secrets for Pain-Free Movement, Maximum Mobility & Flexible Strength
Book By Pavel Tsatsouline
Paperback 130 pages 8.5" x 11"
Over 100 photos and illustrations
#B16 $34.95

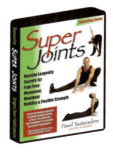

Super Joints
DVD
With Pavel Tsatsouline
Running Time 33 minutes
DVD **#DV003 $24.95**

---

www.dragondoor.com
1-800-899-5111

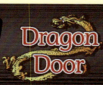

Order *Super Joints* book online:
www.dragondoor.com/B16

Be as FLEXIBLE as You Want to Be—
FASTER, SAFER and SOONER

Relax Into Stretch is for people who want to be flexible and strong, and the principles it will [teach] you can help you stay strong and injury-free in [the] activities of your daily life, not just stretching. [After] a severely herniated lumbar disc a few years [ago,] Pavel's *Power To The People!* was the [beginn]ing of my salvation, *Russian Kettlebell* [Chall]enge taught me to add endurance and some [agil]ity to my strength, and Relax Into Stretch was [the ic]ing on the cake, teaching me how to go from [b]eing able to touch my toes to being able to do [splits] within the space of 6 months while almost 50 [years] old!"—Steve Freides, Ridgewood, NJ

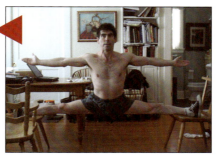

Picture of me in a split - that says it all, and I owe it all to *Relax Into Stretch*. —Steve

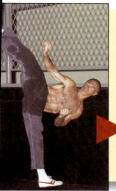

"Pavel has great ideas on flexibility and strength exercises."
—Bill "Superfoot" Wallace, M.Sc., World Kickboxing Champion

The Stretching Bible

"This book tells you HOW and WHY and WHEN to stretch. The photos make it easy to learn the various stretches. This book allows anyone to customize their own stretching program to exactly what their own focus needs to be. I use it as a powerlifter, my wife uses it as a dancer, my boss even used it to get ready to take a ski vacation. A must for every athlete."
—Jack Reape, New Orleans, LA

Stop wasting your stretching time!

"Pavel lines out more information on stretching than I got during the entire 6 years I spent earning a Bachelor's degree in exercise physiology and Master's in physical therapy! The information is clear, easy to read, and works like a charm! I've stretched fairly aggressively over the years with the knowledge I had, but I've made significant gains over the past couple weeks with the information contained on these pages! If you want to do the splits you should get this book!"—Jason Goumas, Lexington, KY

Terrific program—explains all you need!

"A great program for martial arts stretching and stretching for health and wellness. No more back or joint pain. Full leg splits in all four directions within just a few weeks."—Joshua Hatcher, Newington CT, USA

Best stretching book

"When I first read this book, I was 6 inches from doing a full side split and couldn't go down any further. After six weeks of using the principles contained in this book in my own flexibility training, I did my first full side split."—Mercer, NL, Canada

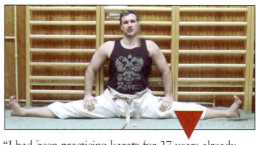

"I had been practicing karate for 27 years already when I learned about Pavel Tsatsouline's stretching books. By that time I totally gave up on a side split. But in these books I read about completely different things, than that I was used to... It took 3 months to achieve my goal ...at the age of 41."
—Dr. Zolnai Vilmos, RKC II, Hungarian Shotokan Karate

- Own an illustrated guide to the thirty-six most effective techniques for super-flexibility
- How the secret of mastering your emotions can add immediate inches to your stretch
- How to wait out your tension—the surprising key to greater mobility and a better stretch
- How to fool your reflexes into giving you all the stretch you want
- Why *contract-relax stretching* is 267% more effective than conventional relaxed stretching
- How to breathe your way to greater flexibility
- Using the Russian technique of *Forced Relaxation* as your ultimate stretching weapon
- How to stretch when injured—faster, safer ways to heal
- Young, old, male, female—learn what stretches are best for you and what stretches to avoid
- Why excessive flexibility can be detrimental to athletic performance—and how to determine your real flexibility needs
- Plateau-busting strategies for the chronically inflexible.

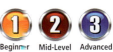

Beginner Mid-Level Advanced

Relax into Stretch
Instant Flexibility Through Mastering Muscle Tension
Book By Pavel
Paperback 150 pages 8.5" x 11"
Over 00 photos and illustrations
#B14 **$34.95**

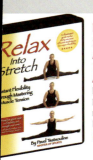

Relax into Stretch
Instant Flexibility Through Mastering Muscle Tension
By Pavel
Running time: 37 minutes
DVD #DV006
$29.95

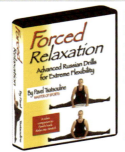

Forced Relaxation
Advanced Russian Drills for Extreme Flexibility
By Pavel
Running time: 21 minutes
DVD #DV007
$24.95

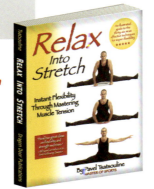

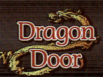

www.dragondoor.com
800·899·5111

Order *Relax into Stretch* book online:
www.dragondoor.com/B14

Instantly—and Measurably!—Increase Your Strength and Power

Go out and test your broad jump or vertical jump. Take three attempts with plenty of rest in between, then rest some and perform a 10sec unique Loaded Stretch developed by one of the top Soviet sports scientists. Jump again. And if you have not broken your record—pack up the DVD and send it back for a quick refund. Only we are not worried, because this instant strength technique is nearly foolproof.

Loaded Stretching techniques work just as well for almost any expression of strength or power, only measuring on the spot may be a more difficult—you are not going to max the deadlift twice in a row! But work it does.

Loaded Stretching is not a flexibility regimen but a specialized strength technique. It is unclear how Loaded Stretching works. Vorobyev (1977) who supervised the research speculated that the external energy applied to the muscle during this special stretch is somehow stored within the muscle chemically. The professor cited the second law of thermodynamics that does not allow for energy to disappear but rather insists on its conversion from one form to another. According to a more recent hypothesis, Loaded Stretching is "static plyometrics" that potentiates the neural wiring of the muscle. But whatever the explanation, LS was shown to instantly increase strength by up to 9.4% and long-term strength gains as well (Efimov, 1977).

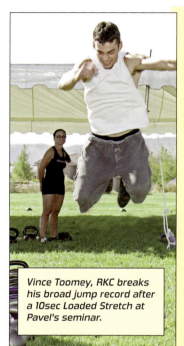

Vince Toomey, RKC breaks his broad jump record after a 10sec Loaded Stretch at Pavel's seminar.

"*Loaded Stretching* can provide everyone an edge.. Pavel leads you thru a series of stretching techniques that can immediately increase stamina. As one approaches their limits, little strength secrets can make the difference between winning and losing. *Loaded Stretching* is that, secrets." —*LOUIE SIMMONS,* Westside Barbell

"The loaded hip stretch using a box, the loaded Russian twist, the loaded RKC clean stretch, and the KB loaded triceps stretch are very powerful tools that I have put in my bag of tricks. The loaded RKC clean stretch has been a real blessing to my football and powerlifting ravaged shoulders. There is a lot more here too for every athlete." —*Jack Reape,* Armed Forces Powerlifting Champion

"It is interesting that we have all these great minds in America, and a tremendous amount of info from the Easter Bloc, but never really entered that special door of duplicating elite performance. It took someone from the Eastern Bloc, to show where the door was. Now he has given the key to that all-important first door to creating elite performance. Pavel's *Loaded Stretching* DVD is that key. Thank You Pavel!" —*Jay Schroeder,* arpprogram.com

Instant Results
"This is definitely different t any other type of stretching done. I followed the protoco on the single hip stretch and was able to perform a solid pistol on the leg that normal gives me trouble. I would highly recommend this DVD anyone that wants an instan increase in strength."—Carl Sipes, RKC, Washington, IL

Striking Power
"I implemented one or two stretches before kicking and punching activity. I did a series of roundhouse kicks. Before the second serie used one of the stretches. The first roundhouse kick went hard and the striking pad smashed into my partner's face." —Taikei Matsushita, RKCII, Tokyo, Japan

Loaded lats for smooth pullups!
"I am a pullup fan and got thi DVD to help with my max. I was very pleased to find that the loaded lats make the first 10 seem like I have "super powers"! I am working back up to 20 reps; I did 19 today. A nice method to learn."
—Gregory W., Portland, OR

- Pull heavier
- Jump higher and farther
- Kick and punch harder
- Squat more
- Throw farther
- Press bigger

Loaded Stretching:
It's not about flexibility.
It's about STRENGTH!

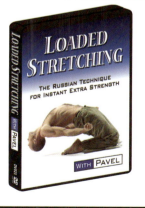

Loaded Stretching
The Russian Technique for Instant Extra Strength
with Pavel
#DV023 $24.95
DVD Running time: 20 minutes

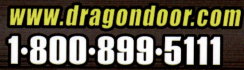

Order *Loaded Stretching* online:
www.dragondoor.com/DV023

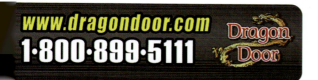

www.dragondoor.com
1•800•899•5111

24 HOURS A DAY
FAX YOUR ORDER (866) 280-7619

ORDERING INFORMATION

Customer Service Questions? Please call us between 9:00am– 11:00pm EST Monday to Friday at 1-800-899-5111. Local and foreign customers call 214-258-0134 for orders and customer service

100% One-Year Risk-Free Guarantee. If you are not completely satisfied with any product—we'll be happy to give you a prompt exchange, credit, or refund, as you wish. Simply return your purchase to us, and please let us know why you were dissatisfied—it will help us to provide better products and services in the future. Shipping and handling fees are non-refundable.

Telephone Orders. For faster service you may place your orders by calling Toll Free 24 hours a day, 7 days a week, 365 days per year. When you call, please have your credit card ready.

Complete and mail with full payment to: Dragon Door Publications, 5 County Road B East, Suite 3, Little Canada, MN 55117

Please print clearly

Sold To: A

Name_____
Street_____
City_____
State_____ Zip_____
Day phone*_____
*Important for clarifying questions on orders

Please print clearly

SHIP TO: *(Street address for delivery)* B

Name_____
Street_____
City_____
State_____ Zip_____
Email_____

Warning to foreign customers:
The Customs in your country may or may not tax or otherwise charge you an additional fee for goods you receive. Dragon Door Publications is charging you only for U.S. handling and international shipping. Dragon Door Publications is in no way responsible for any additional fees levied by Customs, the carrier or any other entity.

Item #	Qty.	Item Description	Item Price	A or B	Total

HANDLING AND SHIPPING CHARGES— FOR MAIL ORDERS ONLY

Phone orders–your Dragon Door representative will give you the exact price
Website orders–shipping and handling will display automatically
Total Amount of Order Add (Excludes kettlebells and kettlebell kits):

$00.00 to 29.99	Add $7.30	$100.00 to 129.99	Add $15.70
$30.00 to 49.99	Add $8.35	$130.00 to 169.99	Add $17.80
$50.00 to 69.99	Add $9.40	$170.00 to 199.99	Add $19.90
$70.00 to 99.99	Add $12.55	$200.00 to 299.99	Add $22.00
		$300.00 and up	Add $26.20

Canada and Mexico double the charges; All other countries triple the charges.

Total of Goods	
Shipping Charges	
Rush Charges	
Kettlebell Shipping Charges	
TX residents add 8.25% sales tax	
MN residents add 7.125% sales tax	
Total Enclosed	

Warning! This may be the last issue of the catalog you receive.

If we rented your name, or you haven't ordered in the last two years you may not hear from us again. If you wish to stay informed about products and services that can make a difference to your health and well-being, please indicate below.

Name_____
Address_____
City_____ State_____ Zip_____
Phone_____

Do You Have A Friend Who'd Like To Receive This Catalog?

We would be happy to send your friend a free copy. Make sure to print and complete in full:

Name_____
Address_____
City_____ State_____ Zip_____

METHOD OF PAYMENT ☐ Check ☐ M.O. ☐ Mastercard ☐ Visa ☐ Discover ☐ Amex

Account No. *(Please indicate all numbers on your credit card)* EXPIRATION DATE CCV

☐☐☐☐ ☐☐☐☐ ☐☐☐☐ ☐☐☐☐   ☐☐/☐☐   ☐☐☐

Day Phone: (___) _____
Signature: _____ Date: _____

NOTE: We ship best method available for your delivery address. Foreign orders are sent by air. Credit card or International M.O. only. For **RUSH** processing of your order, add an additional $10.00 per address. Available on money order & charge card orders only.

Errors and omissions excepted. Prices subject to change without notice.

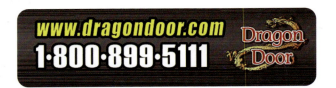

24 HOURS A DAY
FAX YOUR ORDER (866) 280-7619

ORDERING INFORMATION

Customer Service Questions? Please call us between 9:00am– 11:00pm EST Monday to Friday at 1-800-899-5111. Local and foreign customers call 214-258-0134 for orders and customer service

100% One-Year Risk-Free Guarantee. If you are not completely satisfied with any product—we'll be happy to give you a prompt exchange, credit, or refund, as you wish. Simply return your purchase to us, and please let us know why you were dissatisfied—it will help us to provide be products and services in the future. *Shipping and handling fees are non-refundable.*

Telephone Orders For faster service yc may place your orders by calling Toll Free 24 hours a day, 7 days a week, 365 day per year. When you call, please have you credit card ready.

Complete and mail with full payment to: Dragon Door Publications, 5 County Road B East, Suite 3, Little Canada, MN 55117

Please print clearly
Sold To: A

Name_____
Street_____
City_____
State_____ Zip_____
Day phone*_____
* Important for clarifying questions on orders

Please print clearly
SHIP TO: *(Street address for delivery)* B

Name_____
Street_____
City_____
State_____ Zip_____
Email_____

Warning to foreign customers:
The Customs in your country may or m not tax or otherwise charge you an additional fee for goods you receive. Dragon Door Publications is charging y only for U.S. handling and international shipping. Dragon Door Publications is i no way responsible for any additional f levied by Customs, the carrier or any o entity.

Item #	Qty.	Item Description	Item Price	A or B	Total

HANDLING AND SHIPPING CHARGES— FOR MAIL ORDERS ONLY
Phone orders–your Dragon Door representative will give you the exact price
Website orders–shipping and handling will display automatically
Total Amount of Order Add *(Excludes kettlebells and kettlebell kits)*:

$00.00 to 29.99	Add $7.30	$100.00 to 129.99	Add $15.70
$30.00 to 49.99	Add $8.35	$130.00 to 169.99	Add $17.80
$50.00 to 69.99	Add $9.40	$170.00 to 199.99	Add $19.90
$70.00 to 99.99	Add $12.55	$200.00 to 299.99	Add $22.00
		$300.00 and up	Add $26.20

Canada and Mexico double the charges; All other countries triple the charges.

Total of Goods _____
Shipping Charges _____
Rush Charges _____
Kettlebell Shipping Charges _____
TX residents add 8.25% sales tax _____
MN residents add 7.125% sales tax _____
Total Enclosed _____

Warning! This may be the last issue of the catalog you receive.

If we rented your name, or you haven't ordered in the last two years you may no hear from us again. If you wish to stay informed about products and services tha can make a difference to your health and well-being, please indicate below.

Name _____
Address _____
City _____ State ____ Zip ____
Phone _____

Do You Have A Friend Who'd Like To Receive This Catalog?

We would be happy to send your friend a free copy. Make sure to print and complete in full:

Name _____
Address _____
City _____ State ____ Zip ____

METHOD OF PAYMENT ☐ Check ☐ M.O. ☐ Mastercard ☐ Visa ☐ Discover ☐ Amex
Account No. *(Please indicate all numbers on your credit card)*   EXPIRATION DATE   CCV

☐☐☐☐ ☐☐☐☐ ☐☐☐☐ ☐☐☐☐   ☐☐/☐☐   ☐☐☐

Day Phone: ( ) _____
Signature: _____ **Date:** _____

NOTE: *We ship best method available for your delivery address. Foreign orders are sent by air. Credit card o International M.O. only. For **RUSH** processing of your order, add an additional $10.00 per address. Available on money order & charge card orders only.*

Errors and omissions excepted. Prices subject to change without notice.